Ultra Women

Lily Canter and Emma Wilkinson

Ultra Women

The Trailblazers Defying Sexism in Sport

Lily Canter and Emma Wilkinson

Canbury Press

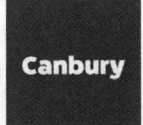

First published by Canbury Press 2025

This edition published 2025

Publisher: Canbury Press (www.canburypress.com)

14 Beresford Rd, London, KT2 6LR, United Kingdom

EU Authorised Representative: Easy Access System Europe

- Mustamäe tee 50, 10621 Tallinn, Estonia, gpsr.requests@easproject.com

Printed and bound in Czechia by Finidr

Typeset in Athelas (heading), Futura PT (body)

FSC® helps take care of forests for future generations.

ISBN:

Paperback 9781914487101

Ebook 9781914487088

Contents

DEFINITIONS

Sex and Gender

The goal of this book is to celebrate women endurance athletes while providing the historical and societal context that has shaped their achievement. We also take a look at the scientific evidence around the factors that may provide female athletes with an advantage. Sometimes we refer to biological sex, other times to gender. By sex we mean the biological difference between males and females that relate to chromosomes, sex organs and endogenous sex hormones. This is not necessarily the same as how someone chooses to identify. We define gender as the socially constructed and enacted roles and behaviours within a historical and cultural context that varies across societies and over time. We have endeavoured to make it clear which we are talking about in a readable way.

Ultra

In the competitive world of running an ultra is defined as any distance longer than a marathon. Meanwhile, sports scientists tend to agree that an ultra-endurance event is a race which takes more than six hours to complete. Since it is possible for some runners to complete an ultra marathon, for example a 50km race, in less than six hours, it is our view that measuring time, rather than distance, appears to be a more reliable and static measure. Therefore, in this book we define ultra sport (whether it is running, cycling, swimming, walking or multisport) as any physical endeavour that lasts six hours or more.

1.
THE AWAKENING

The sun reflected off the frosty moorland which stretched out ahead of her for miles. Stone slabs led all the way down the deserted valley to the Scottish border. Jasmin Paris picked her way down the easterly ridge, using poles to support her shaking legs. With each step a violent shot of pain erupted in her quads, causing her to gently gasp into the crisp air. The burning blisters on her toes and heels, which she had been squeezing to keep herself awake, now brought icy tears to her eyes. Suddenly, she spotted a flash of neon pink as a pig careered through the heather. Shaking her head in disbelief, she continued picking her way down the flagstone path. Minutes later she passed a tree practising the downward dog yoga movement, moments before it transformed into a phosphorescent deer trying to shed its antlers. As she continued step-by-agonising-step along the Pennine Way, Paris passed a waddle of veiled nuns partially shrouded by a row of stone horse heads. She had been running for three days non-stop, covering a gruelling 230 miles, and things were getting surreal.

She was not deterred. 'These visions didn't scare me particularly. I knew at the back of my mind that they couldn't be real and, in some ways, they were a welcome distraction,' she said. That didn't stop her mind from playing tricks on a loop. Disorientated, she flittered between wondering where she was, to panicking that she had gone off course before suddenly realising she was running a race. No ordinary race. Paris was attempting the 268-mile Montane Winter Spine Race for the first time, and she was in it, to win it. The 35-year-old Brit was prepared to take on 50-mile-an-hour winds, freezing January temperatures and 13,300 metres of elevation with little or no sleep. She was travelling on foot from Derbyshire to Scotland with limited daylight hours and checkpoints 50 miles apart. She needed to eat around 10,000 calories a day and carry all of her provisions with her. This was one of the toughest endurance races in the world, and she had just seven days to complete it. On her own. Along an unmarked course. With no support crew. The record at the time, held by Irishman Eoin Keith since 2016, stood at 95:17:00; under four days. Most of the 126 competitors would not complete the race. Did Not Finish rates, known affectionately by athletes as DNFs, reached as high as 60 per cent some years. This was not a race for beginners. The entry requirements indicated that participants should have experience of mountain rescue, extreme mountaineering or the Armed Forces. To the outside world, a new mum who worked full-time treating cats, dogs and conducting research was not the most obvious bet for a podium position. Especially since she needed to stop and express breast milk along the way.

As Paris continued to battle searing pain and unsettling hallucinations, her will was unflinching. She was determined not to let the second-place runner, Eugeni Rosello Solé, from Spain, pass her on the final 38 miles. They had run much of the route together and she was keen to shake him off. 'I'd put so much effort into my Spine preparations, that I wanted an open race. Whilst I know Eugeni was capable of navigating, having run the race several times before, sometimes I felt like a personal guide, leading the way. What probably irked me more, was his assumption that we were running as a team, against the rest of the field – without me ever being consulted.' Believing she could win the race, the mother who had become accustomed to exhausting nights breastfeeding her baby, decided to use sleep deprivation as her final gambit. Though her coach Damian Hall hoped she'd rest and sleep before the race, her inability to do so became her secret weapon.

The reality was that despite her best efforts to wean her 14-month-old daughter Rowan, she was still waking to feed every two to three hours in the night. Paris was not even afforded any respite in her final hours at home, instead enduring a poor night's sleep the Saturday before race day. It didn't matter though, because she was a fell runner who knew how to handle it. Not only was her slim muscular frame attuned to waking in the night to feed, she had years of experience working night shifts as a vet. In a race like this, sleep became highly tactical, especially when you were not the fastest runner in the field. Sleep too much and you would drop places, sleep too little and you'd drop out. At the final checkpoint Paris hedged her bets. 'I most definitely had planned to sleep at Bellingham,' she recalled. 'And yet, when it came to it, I knew that I couldn't. Or at least I couldn't if I wanted to stay ahead and try to win the race. I knew it was a big gamble – at this point I'd been racing for almost three days, with less than three hours of sleep, and I was falling asleep on my feet. But I also knew how hard I'd worked all night staying ahead of Eugeni, and I was fairly certain that if he found me at the checkpoint, he would stick with me to the end... I ate, changed my clothes, drank a strong coffee and left, making my way quickly out of town so that my head torch light wouldn't be seen by the pursuer behind me. It was tough, leaving the warmth and safety of that place, but it helped to know that I was on the last leg, heading for my family, and my bed.'

She stumbled onwards, intermittently falling asleep on her feet before lurching into consciousness. Towards the afternoon as she trudged across the trail it started to get bitterly cold. She stopped in a ditch and put on every item of clothing she had; two pairs of leggings, waterproof trousers, three base layers, one warm layer, a waterproof top plus thick gloves and hat. She tried to move as quickly as possible to stay warm, but every forward leg stretch brought with it a sharp pulling pain up the front of both legs as tendonitis dug deep. Eventually, evening came and with it a dusky shade of pink blending into the cold blue sky. 'It was breathtakingly beautiful, and I was aware even then that the memories of this final ridge run would last me a lifetime. I reached the junction for The Cheviot and paused for a moment, aware of its significance. As I started the descent from Auchope Cairn, the final hints of light retreated and the sky became a deep blue-black, scattered with thousands of stars.' Focused on getting to the finish and seeing her family, she painstakingly hobbled towards a pulsating bright light in the darkness. The last few miles were agonisingly long and the trees lining the road waved their arms at Paris mockingly, tantalisingly human in the silent darkness. Finally, she reached the top of a small rise and saw the village of Kirk Yetholm spread out below her. She started to run, seeing the crowd of lights at the bottom of the green, the voices drawing her in. She was dazzled by a sudden mass of people and flashing lights as she staggered forward and touched the finish line wall. She had won. She had beaten Eugeni Solé. And she had smashed the previous course record by more than 12 hours.

Paris's record was an astonishing 83:12:23. She beat 116 men from 15 countries, in an endurance race where gender didn't matter. Her inspiring achievement became a symbolic tale of the breastfeeding mother who rocked the running patriarchy. Paris spent the next few months in a haze of interviews as journalists across the globe clamoured to cover her story. Her photograph was splashed across national newspapers, she made appearances in Canadian running magazines and her record-breaking story was covered on Australian television. She even made it onto ABC News in America. The peak of her stardom came when the singer Barbra Streisand tweeted: 'What a role model for anyone who believes in rising above the barriers. Jasmin Paris beat her male counterparts by 15 hours and the record by over 12 hours, while pumping breast milk at bus stops! Just amazing. Congratulations, Jasmin! You inspire us all.'

'I wasn't really prepared for the media storm that would result from my run at the Spine,' Paris said later. 'Ironically, the post-race days of family time I'd imagined as I ran were taken over by interviews from all sides, it seemed that everyone wanted to talk to me. While the whole thing was rather overwhelming, I was also touched and deeply inspired by the many messages that I received from women all across the world, telling me their own stories and explaining that I had made a difference to their lives.' It is not surprising that Paris's story captured the public's imagination: it was an incredible achievement, and to the layperson she had battled against all the odds. She had competed in a race where 92 per cent of participants were men. And won. Not by a thin margin. She had shattered the record by half a day. On top of this she was expressing milk at checkpoints whilst being chased down by the previous winner. Paris was one tough mother.

...

To the ultra and fell running communities, however, the race result was no surprise. Insiders knew that Jasmin Paris was the runner to beat. But outside of this enclave, a more sexist narrative prevailed. Society at large assumed that men would always beat women at athletic endeavours. After all, women were physically weaker and not built for such extreme challenges. Suddenly Paris had turned this belief on its head by winning a race outright. It appeared to question everything humanity thought it knew about sport and challenged the patriarchal view of endurance. Paris had demonstrated that at the extreme end of the sport, perhaps women were faster in the long run. Was there something unique about ultra endurance that defied society's expectations of what a woman could achieve? Were women at a physiological and psychological advantage when they were afforded the opportunity to blaze their own trail and test their ultimate limits? Paris had certainly wanted to find out.

Getting up at 5.30am to train near her Scottish home, she worked hard at getting strong. She lived a simple life of running, work and family with no television or social media to distract her. At dawn she could be found dressed in a well-worn running kit, her brown hair tied back into a ponytail, marching her sinewy frame up and down the local ridges. Her commitment to trail running led to wins at the Scottish Hill Running Championships in both 2014 and 2015. Going into the Spine Race she was female British Fell Running Champion despite giving birth to her first child just nine months earlier. In ultra running, she was also making her mark, coming second overall in the six-day Dragon's Back Race in Wales in 2015. Dubbed 'the world's toughest mountain race' the often-treacherous route took in 17,400m of ascent over 220 miles. The summer after her Dragon's Back success Paris ran the Ramsay Round, a craggy circuit of 58 miles and 24 summits including Ben Nevis near Fort William, Scotland, in a time of 16:13, the fastest time recorded for the route. She was also crowned winner of the World Extreme Skyrunning Series the same year and placed sixth female at the 100-mile Ultra-Trail du Mont-Blanc (UTMB), the most competitive ultra marathon event in the world.

So, when the mother-of-one arrived at the start line of the Montane Winter Spine Race in January 2019, she had form. Good form. Described as 'fiercely competitive' by her coach Damian Hall, a fellow Spine race podium finisher, Paris went into the race believing she could win outright. She had enlisted Hall to provide structure and accountability and to 'maximise the potential of the limited free time I had available to train.' One of Paris's huge advantages was her exceptional navigational skills, something she had honed as a hiker. Much of her childhood was spent roaming the mountains of the Šumava National Park in the Czech Republic where her family had a cottage. This continued into her twenties as she spent endless leisurely hours enjoying everything the fells had to offer, before picking up the pace and signing up for her first race in 2008. By the time she won the Spine, 14 years later, with Hall's help, she had mastered her training. She trained every day from October to January in the early hours before dawn by the light of a head torch, mostly in the Pentland and Moorfoot Hills south of Edinburgh. Since her time was limited, weekday runs were capped at 90 minutes maximum, and she fitted in longer runs at the weekend. 'I did my best to fit in with our family plans, so my Saturday long run was often a loop across the Moorfoot Hills to our local parkrun, where I would finish with a fast 5km pushing Rowan in the buggy, whilst Konrad my husband raced for real. My mileage increased gradually, from around 50 miles a week in October, to 100 miles over the New Year, in a week that included three back-to-back long runs of five to six hours each.'

With the exception of her speed sessions, Paris ran everything with a pack, increasing the weight gradually from 1kg to around 6kg by January. To augment the running, she did some strength training, though not as conscientiously as she would have wished. Physical preparation alone was not enough to win the race; Paris needed to be logistically prepared, too. Such is the complexity of the Winter Spine that finishing it, let alone winning it, hinges on carrying the right kit and fuel for up to six days in harsh, snowy conditions. Knowing how tired she would be in the latter stages of the race, Paris laminated a list of essential checkpoint To Dos which included tasks such as 'head torch batteries', 'swap map', 'food and water resupply' and 'breast pump'. Keen to limit checkpoint faffing where chunks of time can disappear without trace, particularly as sleep deprivation sets in, she also prepared food bags for each checkpoint, each one containing the required 3,000 kcals. 'I was determined to be either moving, eating, or sleeping.' Having never run a non-stop race as lengthy as the Spine, Paris was unsure how long it would take. She chose a consistent race pace strategy, one echoed by Sabrina Verjee (whom we will meet in Chapter 14) when she set the Wainwrights outright record in 2021. 'Looking back at the 2018 leaders' splits, it seemed to me that their pace typically started around five miles per hour but dropped to half of that in the later stages,' Paris said. 'I thought a more logical approach would surely be to aim for a steady four miles per hour throughout, with some solid blocks of sleep from checkpoint two or three onwards.'

Out came the laminated list once more as she drew up a colour-coded spreadsheet with split times and rest times for each day, with three extra columns comparing her forecast times with three previous male winners. The strategy worked. Whilst Solé established an early lead, Paris quickly caught him. The pair ran together for almost 200 miles. In the latter, most tiring stages of the race, Paris overtook Solé before pulling ahead of him. This was in large part due to her gamble not to sleep much. While Paris had been happy to run with Solé for sections of the race she was waiting for her moment to strike. She knew she couldn't run faster than him, but she could stay awake for longer. 'I'd had less than three hours sleep in three days and I planned to sleep again at checkpoint four or five but in reality I was in this hot race with Eugeni and I didn't want him to catch me. I knew he would chase me down and probably drop me as he wanted to beat me. He had lain down at the checkpoint and was having a massage and had fallen asleep in the process. This was my opportunity to get away. I had roughly 90 minutes of light and I needed to open as big a gap as possible.' Her actions caused a stir amongst race supporters including a former winner, Pavel Paloncý, who tweeted he was worried she hadn't had enough sleep. Undeterred, Paris decided she would curb her sleep at the final checkpoint despite her plan to power nap. 'I lay down for 30 minutes at checkpoint five, although I couldn't really sleep. I didn't stay longer because I wanted to be out of there before Eugeni arrived.' Her mind was focused. She just had to stay ahead of Solé.

Another tactic that proved invaluable in her strategic arsenal was not underestimating the weather. Temperatures could plunge below zero on the exposed moorlands – it was January, after all – so Paris opted for warmer, but heavier winter clothing, a tactical decision that prioritised warmth over speed. When temperatures plummeted on the exposed tops of the Cheviots she had additional clothing to put on, whilst Solé trailing behind her at this point, suffered irrecoverably from the sudden drop in temperature. He had packed much lighter gear and was unable to get warm. With just 6km to go he pressed his emergency button and was rescued by the support team. 'He had a normal race jacket I would use for summer conditions. I'm not criticising him, you have to take calculated risks. But he had a lot lighter kit and a smaller bag and the problem is if you get really cold you are stuck because you have nothing else to put on.'

Despite it being her first attempt at the Spine, Paris outran and outsmarted all 116 men and the nine other women. She defied the odds, which were assumed to weigh heavily in favour of her male competitors. But then it was her favourite type of race – long, rough, and wild. Fast-twitch muscles, testosterone and lung capacity were not enough. Paris had something else. She trained as hard as the men but had also mastered the art of preparation, navigation and sleep deprivation. 'The longer the race, the more different skills are involved. This race was in midwinter, so it was as much about staying warm, fuelling yourself, the balance between sleep and keeping moving. Then there's the mind stuff and self-belief and the navigation as well. And I think it's one argument as to why women get more competitive than at shorter distances. Maybe they are better at multitasking,' she reflected. Considering everything, it was not surprising that Paris won. Yet the very fact that she was a woman momentarily turned the world upside down. The prevailing wisdom in sport was upended. A woman could outrun a whole field of men by 15 hours.

...

Paris's story is central to understanding how women continue to butt against sexism in sport. In this book we aim to unpick the established view that men are always faster than women. Speaking to scores of endurance experts, we delve into the science of physiology to examine the factors which give women an unexpected advantage. We interrogate claims that women have greater strategy, mental resolve and agility, and we analyse the feats of hikers, runners, swimmers, cyclists and multi-sport racers. But above all, we tell the stories of ultra women who have continued to push back against the male lens in sport. The women who have been denied opportunities, but took them anyway. Because Paris isn't an anomaly. Women across the world have been winning long-distance races outright, and setting ultra-endurance records, for centuries. The world just hasn't been paying attention.

2.
HISTORY MAKERS

Pistols aloft she strode confidently around the rough circular track, one foot in front of the other. From time to time she fired shots into the air to keep onlookers at bay. Nothing was going to stop her. They could try to sabotage her all they wanted, but if she were easily intimidated, she wouldn't be here doing this in the first place. Near the end of her six-week endurance challenge, the bookies were thriving, and thousands had gathered to gawk at her in disbelief. It had turned out to be quite the spectacle, but Emma Sharp never had any doubt she would succeed. She was shaking up her life. Plenty of people, including Sharp's husband, tried to talk her out of her seemingly mad plan. But she was known for being strong-willed. When she set her mind to something she would not be dissuaded. The unusual challenge she had set herself; to walk one mile every hour for 1,000 hours. It was 1864 and 32-year-old Emma Sharp, born and bred in the north of England was ready for an adventure. Something to take her out of the drudgery of the factories and mills she was destined to spend a lifetime in. The one thing she knew she had in spades: stamina.

...

The 'sport' of pedestrianism had begun as an aristocratic pursuit, where gentleman athletes of the day would place wagers on walking feats of great distances. Sometimes they took part themselves, other times they would gamble on the ability of their footmen to walk as they travelled alongside in a carriage. In 1809, a Scot called Captain Robert Barclay Allardice, a well-connected member of the landed gentry, was the first to walk one mile every hour for 1,000 hours for a bet. Over the 42 days it took to complete the event, 10,000 people came to watch. He won 1,000 guineas and the 'Barclay Match' was born. What started out as a gentlemanly show of athleticism over the coming years became a working-class endeavour. Pedestrian events would be held at pubs or showgrounds. It was a way to earn potentially large sums of money from paying spectators and the accompanying gambling. It also became a pursuit that some women realised they were good at. They instinctively knew they could spend many hours on their feet and quickly clocked there was money to be made. Fame too would come from the fact no one expected them to be able to do it. Now 55 years later, Sharp was about to cement her name in history as one of many highly successful female pedestrian walkers who had discovered they had a special talent for the endurance that a Barclay Match – and other long footraces – required.

For Sharp the idea had not come out of the blue. She had read about Margaret Douglas, a mother of seven from Doncaster who had moved to Australia for a better life. Aged almost 40, Douglas had completed several Barclay matches in and around Melbourne, having adopted the mantra 'there is no such word as fail'. Perhaps having exhausted possibilities for earnings in Australia, she was enticed back to England with the promise of £500, the equivalent of more than £52,000 in today's money. For this payday, she would have to walk a mile an hour for 1,000 hours around a wooden boardwalk set up in a theatre in London's Leicester Square. It would take 19 laps to complete a mile circuit, then Douglas would rest on a sofa until the next hour began. She had developed a technique of doing two laps at the end and start of an hour to allow for maximum rest. Posters talked of this 'wonderful feat' where Mrs Douglas would walk 'day and night'. Spectators could pay sixpence to come and watch. In the evening other shows including opera singers and jugglers would occur simultaneously. She was described by onlookers as taking no notice of anyone and monotonously walking lap after lap. Douglas kept her end of the bargain and completed more than 800 miles of the event before the plug was suddenly pulled and the walkway dismantled. The theatre owners accused Douglas of not fulfilling the terms of their agreement. There was a row over the timekeeping book that tracked her efforts. Now out of pocket, she took them to court. A series of hearings never got to the bottom of the disagreement. But the magistrate did not seem convinced that this 'small person of no remarkable powers' could have managed the distance. Nobody had accused her outright of cheating but that was the insinuation. Surely she was deceiving everyone because it wasn't possible for a 42-year-old mother to have achieved such a feat. Needing to recoup her losses later that year, Douglas repeated the challenge, this time at a venue in Liverpool. Vindicated, she completed the 1,000 miles and returned to Australia.

When Emma Sharp read about how Douglas's attempt in London had come to an abrupt end, she declared: 'I could have done that' and immediately made plans, to the horror of her mechanic husband. Sharp had no experience of pedestrianism or race walking. But once the idea formed she wasted no time. Less than two weeks later, she was at the start of a tiny 120-yard track (110 metres) at a local sporting ground in Bradford, West Yorkshire. Unfazed about what she was about to attempt. Sharp convinced the Quarry Gap pub landlord, less than a mile from her home, to host the attraction behind the inn and struck a deal for gate ticket sales. Wearing men's clothing – and without the support of her husband, who found the whole endeavour mightily embarrassing – Sharp did not give much credence to what other people thought. Dressed in a baggy red and black checked jacket and trousers and comfortable boots, she tied her hair up underneath an ornate straw hat. At a quarter to the hour, she set off walking up and down the straight track completing one mile before the hour was up. She went straight into the next mile as the clock ticked into the next hour, to maximise her rest period. In between she retired to her pub room until near the end of the next hour. This continued over the course of six weeks throughout September and October. Sharp was determined to show her grit.

For many of her walks her small dog would happily run alongside her. She was making it look too easy for the gamblers who had come to bet against her. Having never tried anything like this before, wagers were placed in surrounding towns by those who disbelieved a woman could carry this off. Sharp didn't need to train or learn how to be a pedestrian, she just needed belief she would finish what she started. As time went on, interest spread, the crowds grew, and so did Sharp's potential takings. Women in particular seemed to be inspired with the local paper reporting by the time she had done 600 miles no fewer than 5,000 females were watching from the spectators' enclosure. By now it was autumn, the weather had worsened and the rain poured, but still she kept up the same regular speed. Over and over. Those watching could tell she was getting increasingly tired, but Sharp was not a quitter.

Keeping going when she was weary was one thing. But there were many who wanted her to fail, not least the bookies who were set to lose big if she did manage to finish. In desperation, they tried to sabotage her efforts. Repeatedly. Men tried to drug her food, trip her up and disturb her much-needed rest in the short periods when she wasn't walking. In one instance red hot cinders were sprinkled on the track. Sharp continued regardless but the hot coals burned the paws of her canine companion. She told one interviewer covering the spectacle that someone had tried to take her out with chloroform. Yet Sharp shrugged this off and kept going. She armed herself with pistols, one in each hand to protect her safety. Her doggedness generated enough fear of civil unrest that the police were eventually called in to keep the peace. On the final night, an armed officer was sent to walk ahead of her. The last lap – number 14,600 – happened at five in the morning. It is thought almost 20,000 people came to watch her finish with a local brass band playing as she crossed the line. Promising never to do such a thing again, she walked away with at least £500. True to her word, that was her only foray into pedestrianism. She left the mills, took over a grocery shop, and later started a rug business.

...

Across the pond a similar phenomenon was happening in the US with substantial prize money up for grabs. The female pedestrianism craze came in waves in the 1800s. Between 1870 and 1884 there were more than 50 ultra marathon walks completed by more than a dozen female walkers. The best of a very hardy bunch was perhaps Ada Anderson, born in 1843, who became known as the 'Champion Lady Walker of the World'. After trying to make it in the theatre as an actress without much success, she met a British race walker called William Gale who trained her. Anderson prepared for six weeks for her first walk, where she had no more than 20 minutes rest at a time for three weeks. A staggering feat where she used her ability to cope with no or very little sleep to its full advantage. Pretty soon after she broke Barclay's distance record and covered 1,250 miles doing one and a quarter miles at a time. Travelling around the country to push herself to greater extremes, Anderson walked 1,500 miles in 1,000 hours in an event held in Leeds in 1878. Having dominated pedestrianism in the UK, she travelled to the US, to seek her fortune. In 1879, Anderson completed 2,700 quarter miles in the same number of quarter hours at the Mozart Gardens in Brooklyn. The track was so small she needed to do seven laps to complete each quarter mile. Thousands flocked to see her. Ticket sales generated $32,000 with Anderson receiving $8,000 (about $190,000 in today's money). Anderson's superpower was her stunning ability to endure sleep deprivation, on occasion stumbling around as if asleep on her feet, before later becoming alert as if it never happened.

During this period women were also taking part in popular six-day races in America. Among those competing, Amy Howard from Brooklyn stood out. She started her race-walking career at the age of 17. By the end of her first year she had set a new women's world record of 393 miles in the allotted time. Men were still the dominant force in pedestrianism and the women – albeit highly successful – far smaller in number. Despite spectators turning up in their thousands, there were those who thought women's professional walking should be banned. Scuffles would sometimes break out from bystanders who wanted to disrupt the events. In 1880 six-day races, the standard format of pedestrian events at the time, were banned in New York city. The craze which had attracted so much attention was coming to an end. For a while, the determined female racers decamped to the West Coast. Howard was quick so could put distance between her and her fellow competitors and still have time to rest. She won every six-day women's race she entered, despite sometimes offering a head start to the rest of the field. Howard may even have been the first female athlete to be paid for commercial endorsement, promoting Duffy's Pure Barley Malt Whisky which 'relieved the tremendous fatigue after a long match'. She died in childbirth in her early twenties. Her record of 409 miles in six days set in 1881 lasted for 102 years.

...

Over the same time period, another group of intrepid women was taking on the world of mountaineering. Female alpinists. In sharp contrast to the female pedestrians, their long and illustrious history was in part due to their affluence. Writer Rachel Hewitt became interested in the women trailblazers in Alpine adventure after seeing black and white photos of fearless women in long woollen skirts, skating, tobogganing and climbing. Hewitt, author of In Her Nature, went on to discover a band of female explorers leading the way in the 1800s. As climbing gained popularity and clubs were formed to formalise and regulate the sport, women were excluded. They had no choice but to do things on their own terms, going against the norms of the day. At the heart of the story was an upper-class Irish woman, born Elizabeth Hawkins-Whitshed in 1860, but known to her friends as Lizzie Le Blond. Her father, a wealthy landowner, died when she was 11, leaving her a substantial inheritance. Married at the age of 18 and giving birth to her son the year after, Le Blond started spending more time apart from her husband, moving to Switzerland in 1881. Her first climb took her two-thirds of the way up Mont Blanc and by 1907, Le Blond had formed the Ladies Alpine Club. An expert on mountain climbing, she wrote seven books and is credited as one of the first female filmmakers to document women in Alpine activities. The lung problems that had caused her to seek out the therapeutic Alpine air in the first place did not hold her back. Moving to Chamonix for the summer, she scaled Mont Blanc twice.

In her lifetime, Le Blond (Aubrey Le Blond was the surname of her third husband) was the first person – female or male – to ascend 20 mountains. Her photography skills combined with climbing prowess meant she was able to capture views no one had seen before, with hundreds of her photographs formally published. She was achieving firsts at a time when such activities were strongly deemed to be masculine and definitely not for ladies. Le Blond was not alone. The diarist Anne Lister, also known as Gentleman Jack, is primarily remembered as the 'first modern lesbian'. What is less well known is that in 1838, on a trip with her partner Ann Walker, Lister – who was from a wealthy landowning family – was the first person to officially ascend Vignemale (3,298 metres). It took 10 hours for Lister to reach the summit, the highest peak in the French Pyrenees, and another seven to come down again.

Women like Lister and Le Blond were achieving their ambitions in the mountains in relative comfort due to the wealth of their birth; Le Blond had a luxurious tent she would pitch at the foot of a mountain and had staff to help her. They were at the other end of the society to the working-class female pedestrians. But women from all walks of life were keen to test themselves, refusing to be held back by society's expectations. By the 1920s, women had shown they were capable in many areas they had previously been excluded from, largely as a result of the First World War. As men in their millions were drafted to fight in Europe, women took over their jobs in healthcare, agriculture, manufacturing and more. Already popular, women's football took off during this time with around 150 women's football clubs in Britain by 1921. Matches attracted as many as 45,000 spectators. But society was conflicted. There was much debate over whether these were appropriate activities for women to participate in. Might such vigorous activity damage women's health? The English Football Association (FA) took note and banned the women's game from professional grounds in 1921 because it was 'quite unsuitable for females and ought not to be encouraged'. But plenty of women remained resolutely defiant in the face of societal pressure. Women who set themselves challenges that many thought were unacceptable for their gender.

Two years after the FA banned women's football, an intrepid group of five no-nonsense women set out to compete in a very different sort of endurance race. One that only women could do. In fact, only women with babies. An ultra race with prams, proposed by Ada May Edwards, a 32-year-old Manchester mother of six. Edwards put an advert in the Derby Daily Telegraph for 'any mother of three or more living children' to take part in a pram race from London to Brighton. The rule was they had to push their youngest child who must be under six months old, 'in a perambulator' for the 52-mile distance. The winner would get £6. It was a controversial event that attracted threats of legal action and protests from the National Society for the Prevention of Cruelty to Children. Undeterred, Lily Groom, Rose Firmager, Alice Sunderland, Margaret Oliver and Ada May Edwards lined up outside Big Ben in Westminster, in the heart of the capital. Fuelled with chocolates, oranges and tea, every one of them completed the distance, stopping on the way to feed their babies, who were wrapped up against the cold. Thousands of spectators watched as the women, dressed in corsets and heavy woollen clothing, reached the end in Brighton. The winner of the double marathon was Groom who completed the route in 12 hours and 20 minutes.

...

Walking was not the only endurance endeavour women took part in long before official ultra races were conceived. Despite women's professional cycling barely existing until the 1990s, female cycling pioneers can be traced back to the 1800s. Louise Armaindo, a Canadian strongwoman, trapeze artist and race walker, was one such woman who took part in penny-farthing bicycle races. In 1886, she held the record for the longest distance in a multi-day indoor cycling event of 843 miles. She had been a pedestrian walker before moving to the 'high wheel' bike and she wasn't the only one. Annie Londonderry (or Annie Cohen Kopchovsky to use her real name) was a Jewish Latvian immigrant who reportedly became the first woman to ride around the world, setting off on her sponsored journey in 1894. Meanwhile, Alfonsina Strada caused a stir in 1924 when she managed to enter the annual Giro d'Italia after being mistaken for a man. Her participation in the multi-stage event whipped up so much publicity organisers allowed her to compete. Described as a 'devil in a dress' by newspaper reports, Strada was beset with problems following a crash which damaged her bike. Of the 90 cyclists who started, she was among 38 riders who made it to the end. She went on to win 36 races against men during her illustrious career.

While alpinism and cycling were seen to belong to realms of men, a more acceptable leisure pursuit for women in the 1900s was swimming. In 1926, a story on the northern coast of France seized the public's attention. During the summer, five young women attempted to become the first to swim the English Channel. This was not the fairly routine challenge it is now. At the time only five men had ever made it across the 21-mile-wide sea separating England and France. Not only were the women taking on the unpredictable tides and weather, jellyfish and shipping lanes, they had to make their own swimwear that could both withstand the rigours of the challenge and not actively hamper them. To help make it possible, they crafted homemade goggles to keep the seawater out. The challenge across the choppy cold waters was notoriously difficult. A Frenchwoman, Jeanne Sion had abandoned an attempt in 1922 after 14 hours of swimming. Clarabelle Barrett, a 35-year-old swimming teacher from the US, also failed in the summer of 1926 when the media was gripped by multiple attempts. Seen as a courageous outsider, the six-foot-tall Barrett – who had no financial backing – had to be taken out of the water with exhaustion in thick August fog, after swimming for 21 hours. The Daily Mail described it as the 'finest' swim ever accomplished by a woman. A long-distance swimmer from Boston in the US, Eva Morrison, also took part that summer, making the first of three unsuccessful attempts.

One of the most promising swimmers was Lilian Cannon, a 23-year-old American, who had gained fame by swimming 12 miles across the Chesapeake Bay, the largest estuary in the United States. Public interest in her ability increased when a young man, George Lake, who had been swimming across the Bay alongside Cannon, had to be pulled from the water, exhausted, at the halfway point. Cannon had no such trouble and completed the Chesapeake challenge with relative ease. With the backing of her local newspaper, the Baltimore Post, Cannon tried twice to cross the Channel but was thwarted first by a terrible storm, then stomach cramps. At the same time, Mille Gade, a Danish-American mother of two, was also preparing to take on the sea between England and France, financed by a wealthy businessman. Gade had already made the newspapers back home by swimming 42 miles around Manhattan Island and being only the second person – and the fastest – to swim the 153 miles from Albany to New York.

But Gade was beaten to the record by a 20-year-old, Gertrude Ederle. By the time she stepped into the water at Cape Gris Nez, Ederle was already a US and world record holder and Olympic gold medallist. She had aborted an attempt to swim the Channel the previous summer, exiting the water at Kingsdown in Kent after swimming 35 miles in 14 hours and 34 minutes. In 1926, she became not only the first woman to cross the Channel but the fastest person by two hours, beating a time set by Enrique Tirabocchi of 16 hours 33 minutes. Her achievement created waves back home in the US. Ederle had been signed up by the Chicago Tribune to write a column on her attempt as well as receiving backing from the New York Daily News. Such was the excitement and publicity generated by Ederle's success that when the 'Queen of the Waves' returned to New York she was greeted by a ticker-tape parade in her honour and cheered by two million people. Ederle's record stood until 1951 and is still remembered today with her achievement making it onto the big screen in the Disney film, Young Woman and the Sea.

These swimming pioneers were undoubtedly breaking waves through their tenacity and innovation. They made their own kit, found sponsors, and enlisted local experts to help them navigate treacherous currents. They set records that stood for decades. Now, a century later, women are still breaking, holding and building on those records. In 2019 Sarah Thomas became the first person to swim four times across the English Channel non-stop. The US swimmer had already set the record for the longest lake swim two years earlier after covering 168.3 km (104.6 miles) in 67 hours and 16 minutes at Lake Champlain on the border between New York and Vermont.

...

Throughout history, countless women have challenged the limits of what was believed possible for them to achieve physically. The defiant and determined individuals mentioned above are but a snapshot. Despite showing they had the ability to excel in endurance, women were still seen as weaker and unable to manage such taxing physical endeavour. Most of them were told they couldn't or shouldn't be doing these feats – but they did them anyway. Society deemed that none of this was 'ladylike.' Yet those who were most determined managed to forge their own path. They proved they could hold their own in these more obscure and unusual challenges. But this didn't stop the exclusion. As sport became more popular, and governing bodies formalised the rules, women were continually told they weren't as physically capable as men. Despite the wealth of history demonstrating otherwise, they had to fight to take their place. One particular race exemplifies this most starkly. A race that hundreds of thousands of women participate in every year, but which for many decades was seen as too dangerous for females to even attempt.

3.
MARATHON EFFORT

She wouldn't take no for an answer. The world had gathered for the inaugural modern Olympic Games and only men were allowed to compete. A new event had been devised as the pinnacle of sporting prowess. The marathon would be the crowning glory of this celebration and Stamata Revithi wanted to be a part of it. The poverty-stricken young mother begged organisers to do it. This could be her big break. But her appeals fell on deaf ears. Her response? She did it anyway.

Ancient Greece had been the inspiration for the modern Olympics. Every four years from 776 BC, any free Greek man could put themselves forward to take part in boxing, running and chariot racing among other events. It was this male-only contest that influenced the French aristocrat Pierre de Coubertin to revive the spectacle in 1896. And of course, women would not be allowed. They never had been. In ancient Greece, there had been another festival held every four years that celebrated the athletic achievement of female competitors. During the 'Heraea,' young unmarried girls took part in footraces, in different age categories, to honour the Greek goddess Hera. Competitors wore a short loose piece of cloth tied over one shoulder with one breast exposed, as shown by a marble statue from 560BC now in the British

Museum. A committee of women oversaw the Heraea and winners were given a crown of olive leaves. None of this swayed the organisers of the modern Olympic Games when they banned all women from not only competing, but also entering the stadium to watch. Pierre de Coubertin was stridently against women taking part in any Olympic event. The pervasive view that women were frail and physically weak was particularly prevalent among the aristocratic circles that de Coubertin moved in. In the 1800s, the dominant 'medical' opinion was that women had a fixed amount of energy, meaning they could not do both physical and intellectual tasks. As a result, women had been excluded from most activities since the dawn of competitive sport.

It meant nothing to Stamata Revithi, a blonde, thin mother of a young child, who looked much older than her 30 years. Having enjoyed long-distance running in her youth, she saw the marathon as a way to gain fame and money, or at least employment. After living in poverty in Piraeus, Greece, she desperately needed a new start. Her elder child had recently died at the age of seven. Newspaper reports suggest she would travel around on foot with her baby in her arms. After a fellow traveller told her to run in the marathon to turn her fortunes around, the plan became set in her mind. Revithi was strong, she could endure and she had stamina, often having to survive on little food and going to bed hungry. Revithi went to the committee and asked to enter. The answer was a resounding no, with the reason given that she had missed the deadline.

Revithi shrugged her shoulders and declared she would run anyway, caught a cart to the small village of Marathon and revelled in her newfound fame as journalists jostled to interview her. Described by the historian Athanasios Tarasouleas as a vibrant and clever woman, she told the throng of reporters peppering her with questions that she would compete even if it was not official. She would just follow behind. 'I saw in a dream that I had an apron full of gold and gilded sugared almonds' she said before continuing 'my heart is in it, I suppose my feet will hold'. Another runner who said everyone would have gone home by the time she finished, was given short shrift by Revithi and told not to 'demean women'. Journalists asked how she would sustain herself on the route and she told them she had no plans to eat, something she was used to. While she did not join the male marathon runners, she did run it the next day, starting at 8am and asking local officials including the mayor to record the time. Revithi completed the route in five and a half hours, begging a group of officers for signatures to prove the time of her arrival. When they asked the sweaty and dusty runner why she had done it she answered 'so the King might award a position to my child'. She then declared she was off to see Timoleon Philimon, secretary general of the Greek Olympic Committee, to tell him of her achievement.

What happened to Revithi has been lost to history. Reports are mixed and further complicated by the fact that sometimes she is referred to as Melpomeni. Some accounts have her completing the marathon as a trial run and eating oranges along the way. Whatever the circumstances, Revithi is widely acknowledged to have been the first woman to run the inaugural modern Olympic marathon, even if her achievement has never been formally recognised.

In those first modern Olympic Games there were around 241 participants and none of them were women. De Coubertin argued that it would be a logistical headache to set up separate events, that it was inappropriate to watch women compete with each other – and that the female sex had limited physical abilities.

De Coubertin's unyielding views were not uncommon in the 19th century. In polite society women's athletics was considered to be centred around graceful movement rather than strenuous competition. The committees overseeing organised sporting events were backed by the doctors of the time who believed intense physical exercise was dangerous for women. Pseudo-scientific explanations focused on menstruation as being a 'particular burden' for women, leaving them with a finite amount of physical and mental energy.

On both sides of the Atlantic the popular medical opinion was that having a period was essentially an illness which needed to be managed through avoidance of vigorous activity. Energy needed to be conserved rather than used up in overtaxing competition. Too much running might cause a uterus to fall out. Women's primary role was to have babies and this had to be protected. This became something of a self-fulfilling prophecy. Middle-class women in particular followed the expectations around wearing restrictive clothes, eating little and exercising even less. 'Not surprisingly, they would often faint, become ill and behave submissively, thus confirming the medical stereotype of the 'delicate' female,' noted the sports sociologist Jennifer Hargreaves.

In line with these views, de Coubertin decreed that allowing women to participate in the Olympics would be 'impractical, uninteresting, unaesthetic and incorrect'. It was strictly a celebration of male athleticism and physical prowess. The marathon was the most strenuous of them all. Testing competitors to their limits. Named after its starting location, the race involved competitors running 40km from Marathon to Athens. Only the fittest and strongest of men could complete such an event. The accomplishments of women during the pedestrianism craze of the 19th century (see Chapter 2) were brushed aside. The belief that women could not handle endurance activities persisted into the 20th century, maintaining the status quo. The notion that women could not cope with anything other than the shortest running events was further cemented on a single day at the 1928 Olympic Games in Amsterdam. Women had been allowed to enter swimming and tennis events in 1908 and 1912. At the 1928 Games, the organisers reached a deal with the International Federation of Women's Sports for women to take part in track and field events for the first time. The federation had responded to de Coubertin's refusal to let women into the Olympics by setting up its own popular version and continuing to lobby hard for acceptance. In Amsterdam, nine women ran in the 800-metres – all of them finishing. A new world record of two minutes and 16 seconds was set by Germany's Karoline

Lina Radke. Afterwards, as some of the women lay on the grass beside the track exhausted (unsurprisingly, as they had been trying to keep up with a world record pace), the watching media took this as a sign that women were indeed too fragile to participate. Over-excited newspapers in the US, UK and Canada reported that women had collapsed after the race; evidence that 800 metres was too strenuous and beyond women's capabilities. Claims were made that women would be desexed and their reproductive abilities impaired by the exhaustion. The International Olympic Committee agreed, stating that the 800-metre distance was too hard for women after all. De Coubertin himself said this had 'justified my opposition to allowing women into the Olympic Games'. The position held for decades and the women's 800-metres only reappeared in 1960.

Between the first and second world wars, there remained a great deal of hostility to female athletics. The ideology that women were not capable of serious athleticism or would even harm themselves remained persistently stubborn even in the face of proof that women could compete. In 1926, an Englishwoman called Violet Piercy ran the London Olympic marathon course – unofficially – in a stunning time of three hours 40 minutes, although with some debate about whether the full distance was covered. Later becoming known as one of the first female endurance runners in Britain, Piercy would continue to run lengthy distances. She ended up with an official women's Windsor to London marathon time of four hours 25 minutes as part of a men's race. Proof it could be done. It did not matter that she had run the distance without any apparent ill effects. Commentators at the time still argued that athletics were unsuited to a woman's physique and thus harmful to the properties of motherhood.

The opposition to women participating in longer endurance events stuck to such an extent that by 1966, when Roberta Gibb, known as Bobbi, applied to run the Boston Marathon she was refused on the grounds that 'women are not physiologically capable of running a marathon'. The dismissive letter from the race organisers struck her as outrageous, especially given she was already running up to 40 miles at a time. Like Revithi 70 years earlier and Piercy four decades before, her reaction was 'to hell with them' and she made a plan to run anyway. With no official coach, Gibb had spent the summer training in secret while travelling around the country in a VW Camper Van. On the day of the race, her mother drove her to the start from their home on the outskirts of Boston with her father refusing to help. Wearing shorts over a swimsuit and a large hooded sweatshirt, she hid in the bushes before joining the crowd of runners after the race began. Gibb quickly got too hot but was worried about taking her jumper off and revealing her identity. In a show of solidarity, the men running near her said they would not let her be thrown out and so she ran freely. When she passed Wellesley College, a famous female-only university, a great cheer went up. She finished in three hours, 21 minutes, 40 seconds, despite being in pain from wearing a pair of men's trainers that rubbed her feet.

Gibb also ran unofficially the next year, as did another famous pioneer of female running, Kathrine Switzer. Switzer became known as the first woman to officially finish the Boston marathon in 1967 because her application had slipped through the net. Boston is one of the oldest marathon races, itself inspired by those first official Olympics, and with its inaugural race in 1897. Yet despite the stringently applied no-women rule, there was no mention of gender in the rule book. When Switzer was formulating her plan to enter, she was aware that the Amateur Athletic Union (AAU) had limited women's races to no longer than a mile and a half. This was an era when women's races generally covered no more than 800 metres. In the swinging sixties, women were pushing back against the social limitations they were under. Yet for female runners, there were still no opportunities to prove they could in fact take on longer distances. Signing up to the Boston event with just the initials KV Switzer, her entry seemed to go unquestioned rather than being immediately rejected as Gibb's had been.

The black and white photos of Switzer running in a plain grey tracksuit, the official 261 race number pinned to her chest, have now been reproduced in many articles discussing the rise in popularity of women's running. The photos are extraordinary not for how they highlight the evolution of running kit but because they capture the moment in which Switzer is tackled by the race director Jock Semple, who was apparently known for charging after participants not following the rules. At the start of the race, the 20-year-old Switzer, who was running with her coach and boyfriend, had the hood of her sweatshirt up to counter the cold snowy New England weather. It was only once the race was well underway that organisers realised there was a woman on the course with an official number, which Semple immediately tried to rip off her front.

In her memoir, Marathon Woman, Switzer recalled that the previous year she rowed with the coach of the men's cross-country team. She had been forced to join because there was no women's running equivalent in New York, where she was a journalism student. Despite seeing Switzer running 10 miles a night in training, Arnie Briggs was insistent that a marathon distance would be too much for a woman to handle. They made a deal that if she ran 26 miles in practice, he would take her to Boston to compete for real. Just to really hammer home her point, Switzer ran 31 miles in that trial run.

At the starting line, other runners noticed a woman in their midst but were welcoming and friendly, just as they had been to Gibb the year before. But a couple of miles in when the photo press truck passed them, a man in an overcoat ran over and started remonstrating, pulling her glove off in the process. This was closely followed by a furious Semple screaming 'get the hell out of my race' at Switzer, who was embarrassed and fearful. Briggs tried to push Switzer away. Switzer's boyfriend, an ex-American football player called Tom Miller, shoved Semple to the side and the group ran fuelled by adrenaline as the press chased a now terrified Switzer. Over those long miles Switzer's fear turned to anger, knowing that if she quit 'no one would believe that women had the capability to run 26-plus miles'. She crossed the finish line in four hours and 20 minutes.

In an almost perfect example of the barriers that women were up against, Boston Athletic Association and the Amateur Athletic Union, despite now being faced with two years of proof that women could in fact run the marathon successfully, doubled down. Where there had been no mention of gender, they brought in new rules barring women from all competitions with male runners. It took until 1972 for an official women's race to be established as part of the Boston marathon and in 1974, Switzer was the female winner of the New York City marathon. Her personal best came the following year in Boston with a time of two hours 51 minutes.

The decades-long deeply embedded opinion that women should not take part in longer races meant that women were not allowed to compete in the Olympic marathon event until 1984. When the 50 female competitors lined up on the starting line in Los Angeles, Switzer was on hand to mark history as a race commentator. It was a hot August day but the winner, US runner Joan Benoit, took the lead from mile three and held on to the end, completing the event in two hours and 24 minutes. It was watched around the world and was linked to a boom in women's road running in subsequent years. Women's running had finally moved into the mainstream, 88 years after that first Olympic marathon run by a penniless young Greek mother dressed in rags. For women, the marathon was just the start. Some were running much further and not just on the road or track. They were taking on tricky and remote terrain. Running ever more extreme events. Quietly behind the scenes, away from the TV cameras, a small group of spirited women were creating waves in ultra sport, taking on long runs on the trails and mountains, to showcase their inner steel.

4.
GOING THE DISTANCE

There had been weeks of earnest discussion about whether a woman should be allowed to take part in such a brutal endeavour. Back and forth the debate went. Some competitors were on her side but the organisers were worried. Now with just a week to go the green light had finally been given and she would take her place alongside 47 men. A group of elite athletes about to emulate the most legendary of running feats. When Eleanor Adams (now Eleanor Robinson) lined up at the inaugural Sparthalon ultra marathon on 30th September 1983 she had not been able to prepare in the same way as the others. The decision to let her run in the 153-mile race had been so last minute. The gruelling race ahead was made even more daunting by the tight cut-off times that could see her thrown out if she couldn't keep up.

This small group of runners was attempting to recreate the fabled journey of Pheidippides, the running messenger dispatched to Sparta to fetch help when the Persian army landed in Marathon in Greece in 490BC (a distance of 150 miles). As the traditional tale goes, he covered the distance in about a day and a half, ran back again, and then managed another 25 miles to the battlefield (which inspired the marathon race), before finally going back to Athens to announce the Greek victory, when he promptly collapsed and died. How much is accurate – the ancient historian Herodotus does mention an Athenian messenger sent to secure help – and how much has been romanticised in the telling, has long been up for debate. Whether entirely true or not, Pheidippides' feat is the reason why so many runners lace up their trainers to put themselves through a marathon distance. For anyone who has ever wondered why a marathon is such a random 26.2 miles, the British royal family wanted the race at the 1908 Olympic games to start on the lawn of Windsor Castle so the committee added on a bit to make sure it finished in the Olympic Stadium.

The Spartathlon ultra race, also inspired by Pheidippides' epic journey, began as a preliminary expedition by the military. Eleven experienced long-distance male runners from the Royal Air Force were dispatched to explore the route that the running messenger may have taken 2,500 years earlier. The task of this highly trained team of men was to test whether the journey could be done on foot in two days. Three of the 11 managed to finish the 150-mile journey in under 39 hours. It was enough of a success that an official Spartathlon race was deemed possible. Robinson was fairly new to ultra running having only completed her first event – a 12-hour race round a track – the previous summer. She was good, that much was apparent from the start. When she was a 14-year-old girl competing on the track, women weren't allowed to run distance races. To be fair, men weren't overly encouraged to run distance races either, with such strict time cut-off times that it was a fairly elite sport by default. By the 1980s, this competitive environment remained and extended to ultra running, which meant few individuals, and even smaller numbers of women, made their way to the starting line. Robinson's break into ultra running came almost by accident after a race in Nottingham near her home caught her attention. 'I hadn't heard of 100k races or anything like that, it was something I discovered quite by chance and I found I was quite good at it.' In that first 12-hour race, which she chose to do because it meant she could watch her three small children playing nearby as she ran, she broke three world records.

Over the next year she competed in a 100k track race and three 24-hour races. Just two months before Spartathlon, she took part in the Charles Rowell Six Day Track Race in Nottingham, setting a world best of 659km. 'Gradually one or two of us [women] came on the scene and in a sense, I look on myself as a pioneer, opening up the way to all these floods of people now who are having a go and can run for the pleasure of it. People are encouraged to do it, whereas in my day we weren't at all and the Spartathlon is a prime example of that. We were celebrating Pheidippides doing his run and he was a soldier and male so questions were asked, why do we need women in this sport?' In the end it was her male colleagues who convinced the organisers to let her run, but the very last-minute decision left her no time to train or prepare beyond the running she normally did. In a sense she was starting on the back foot. 'It was a case of just turn up and go.'

The Spartathlon is described as the 'world's most gruelling race' with a course that takes participants over rough terrain, through olive groves, up steep rocky hillsides and a mountain section without a path run in the middle of the night. In general, only around a third of those who start the race finish. These days it is a well-oiled machine, with clear pre-race information and briefings, regular aid stations and medics on hand. Of the 379 registered entrants for the 2023 race, 28 per cent were female. But for Robinson, there were no aid stations: 'The most you had was a bottle of water left at the side of the road and if you were near the back of the pack there may not have been any left by the time you got there.' Most people had some sort of support crew with them to meet them at certain points and provide a drink but the information they had to help them to find their way and meet their runner was limited. In some of the villages they passed there would be few random snacks set out on a table. The most terrifying part was running up and over Mount Parthenion in the dead of night, scrambling up over steep, rocky terrain. 'Going up the mountainside in the dark, we had to equip ourselves with torches and you could look behind you and see all these little lights climbing up. It was really quite scary if you thought about it, you just didn't let yourself.' She remembers the runners didn't really mind the lack of organisation (the coach trip of the course the previous day to prepare the runners and their crews had got lost six times), the heat, or the strict time limits, it was just a thrill to be involved. 'We just accepted we were in Greece running this historic event and it was great to be doing it.'

Even the most experienced ultra runner can never be completely sure at the start of a race if they are in fact going to finish – and this challenge was a particularly unknown entity for all involved. 'It's part of the attraction I suppose. In a sense everyone is on a level playing field because you just don't know what's going to happen. I've been in races where I've had to pull out due to stomach issues throwing up at the side of the road, others where I've been totally dehydrated. You could easily stumble over something in the dark so you're never confident, you just go step by step.' After running for 32 hours and 37 minutes in hot weather, beating the cut-off times despite the dreaded stomach problems that every ultra runner fears, she reached Sparta cheered on by enthusiastic well-wishers pressing flowers into her hands as she crossed the square, climbed the steps and touched the statue of King Leonides. She was the ninth runner to finish among those who made it to the end. 'I don't recall being marked out as anything special, everyone who finished was given the same welcome.' She refused offers to take her to hospital to get checked and just sat on the steps of the statue until she felt better. 'I was just euphoric, I'd not only finished but I'd finished in front of some very good runners. I was only just getting to grips with the fact I was quite good at this.'

With the benefit of hindsight, it was always apparent that endurance may have been Robinson's special skill. Running round the streets as a small child in Middlesbrough in the north of England, the remaining bomb craters from the Second World War a perfect playground for her band of friends, she knew she would never win a sprint race – from one end of the street to the other – but set off round the block and she would easily keep going when everyone else had tired and given up. 'I knew from a very early age that the further I went, the better I was compared with everybody else.' Convincing her teachers that longer events were her forte, she ended up representing Yorkshire at the English Schools Track and Field Championships with half a mile the furthest the girls were allowed to run. Then later, a running boom in the 1980s brought with it the concept of the People's Marathon in Birmingham where anyone could have a go. Training for it at night when her very small children were asleep, she surprised herself on race day with a time of three hours 20 minutes. It was a race that has been credited with lighting the spark of Britain's love of mass long distance events. For Robinson, that marathon was just the start. It led to a lengthy and stunningly accomplished career in which she broke almost 40 world records running everything from 30 to 1,000 miles. It wasn't until a broken hip five years ago (six weeks before a World Duathlon Championship she was training for) that she began to slow down a bit. Now an energetic 76-year-old she regularly competes in half marathons. Throughout it all she has been motivated simply by curiosity: 'I just wanted to know what I could achieve.'

That curiosity took Robinson to the starting line of another inaugural road race that has now become legendary among ultra runners. Badwater in California is very hot and very dry. There is a reason the area is known as Death Valley. About 146 miles to the west is the peak of Mount Witney – the tallest in the US and known to be zero degrees in the middle of summer. Races rarely get more extreme than this. By the 1980s, dozens of runners had attempted the crossing which goes from 86 metres below sea level to 4,417 metres above. Despite many attempts at the distance, by 1987 only seven men and one woman had completed it and the route had never been raced. In 1986, an intrepid band of ultra runners planned an official race from Badwater to Mount Witney but cancelled at the last minute because of a lack of liability insurance. Nonetheless the seed was sown and a year later, an Englishman and American had a wager which pitted two male-female running teams against each other in a Badwater contest. Robinson, then aged 39, had plenty of ultra experience under her belt including being the first woman to bust through 200 miles (322km) in a 48-hour race. To get her place at Badwater, she had answered an advert in Athletics Weekly placed by Ken Crutchlow, the Brit who made the bet. Known as an adventurer and entrepreneur, Crutchlow had already taken on feats that included hitchhiking around the world, racing to the top of the Empire State Building and cycling from Los Angeles to Mexico. It was a stroke of genius teaming up with Robinson, who with her ultra running credentials was favourite to win – and her US competitor Tom Crawford knew it. 'We're running against the greatest ultra runner in the world. I don't see Eleanor as the greatest woman ultra runner, she's the greatest ultra runner. Eleanor is the epitome of the greatest athlete in the world,' Crawford told journalists. But Robinson had one huge disadvantage – she trained in the temperate British climate and had no experience of running in 45-degree Celsius heat or racing at altitude.

Nonetheless, she was resolute: 'I never thought I wouldn't do it, it's there to be done,' she said. In the end, the temperature and altitude were 'just another thing' to overcome. She led the race, extending a seven-minute lead to almost six hours by ploughing on steadily through the night. She reached the top of Mount Witney after 52 hours 45 minutes just before a hailstorm struck. It was a new women's record and beat the previous course record by three hours. The US team, which featured Crawford and Jean Ennis finished in 58 hours while an out-of-shape Ken Crutchlow, the man who started the whole endeavour, got to the top of Mount Witney after more than 126 hours. Robinson wasn't doing it to win a bet, this was just another test of her endurance mettle. 'I just went into it to do the best I could. The grudge match was nothing to do with me.' Now known as the Badwater 135, the race stops 11 miles short of where Robinson triumphed but still covers three mountain ranges on the way. For the 46th anniversary in 2023, 100 athletes from 26 countries took part, including 40 women.

Ashley Paulson, aged 41, broke the female course record with a time of 21 hours 44 minutes.

...

While road running was becoming increasingly popular in the 1980s, a handful of women in the UK were already making their mark on the fells. Those in the know will tell you that fell runners are a different breed. A quintessentially British sport, fell running is not the same as trail, off-road or cross country. In the mountains (or fells) a compass is vital. Navigation skills are a must. Paths can be vague or non-existent and it's part of the fun to find the best route. There's a lot of climbing and to witness a fell runner in full pelt on the way down a steep hillside is to know they are not to be trifled with. From the start, this adventurous sport was dominated by men. But it was perhaps more equal than other running pursuits. Women weren't banned as they had been in road marathons. They were allowed, and a handful of them took up the opportunity. Wendy Dodds did her first Karrimor International Mountain Marathon (later rebranded as the Original Mountain Marathon) in 1972 after a friend in the university orienteering team suggested they give it a go. The previous year, a couple of women with a background in 'scrambling' had started the event but not completed it. Dodds and her teammate, Val Pacey, became the first women to finish the two-day race, that year held in the Scottish Borders and designed to test orienteering skills to the limit. Another woman, Debbie Gale completed it as part of a mixed pair with her husband. Still going strong today, the event is a double marathon in which pairs carry all the kit they need to camp overnight (there is a compulsory list). They must be completely self-sufficient and competitors are only told the route once the race begins. There are now six different classes of competition varying in length and severity. In the early 1970s, there were just two – elite and class A. For a few years, Dodds ran in a mixed team, but she soon realised she preferred running as a women's pair because of the camaraderie and generally having 'a good laugh'.

It was an era when walkers, fell runners and others were conjuring up ever more impressive ultra challenges. Ten years into her fell running career, Dodds became the first person to ever complete the Paddy Buckley Round in the Welsh mountains. In this male-dominated sport, the small numbers of women who were participating showed that they were equal to the task. Named after the man who devised the route (but never ran it himself), the Buckley is a circuit of 61 miles (100km) that takes in 47 summits including Yr Wyddfa (Snowdon). Dodds describes Buckley as a great friend – they met doing mountain marathons – and she was dragged along to go on recces of this new challenge he had devised. Three of them started, including Buckley and another man called Bob Roberts, but both Buckley and Roberts bailed. It seemed they did not have Dodds' stubbornness to finish what she started. She carried on alone with only the odd 'navigational hiccup' for more than 24 hours – outside the target they had set themselves. She was fairly confident she could finish the challenge, having been the fourth woman to complete a Bob Graham Round, the equivalent 24-hour challenge over 66 miles (106km) in the English Lake District. Buckley had tried to convince Dodds to stop doing the Paddy Buckley Round and try again another time. Determined to finish, especially after various false starts thanks to the notoriously unpredictable Welsh weather, Dodds stopped worrying about time and just kept on going. 'I always tend to be stronger towards the end. I haven't much speed but I knew intuitively from my swimming days I was better at longer distances.' Her ability to endure over long distances, keeping going when others had quit was not her only advantage. Like Jasmin Paris, who hit the headlines after her Spine record (see Chapter 1), Dodds felt at home in the hills. She spent a couple of years working in Scotland near the Cairngorms and every free weekend was spent exploring. In addition to her navigational skills, she was good at keeping a steady pace. Psychologically that was a good place to be, she said, in the type of events where experience counts for a lot. 'Some people might think it's bad to be at the back of the pack earlier on, but it's nice to work your way through as people start to struggle later on.'

Dodds, who worked full-time as a doctor, was also among those making history at the inaugural Dragon's Back race in 1992. The first major stage race in the UK, with competitors covering the brutal mountains of Wales over five days, she was part of the only women's pair taking part, alongside Sue Walsh. They came ninth. Twenty years later, she did the race again and this time she was the oldest finisher ever. Her story sits alongside another legendary fell runner who was also pushing boundaries at the dawn of UK ultra-running events. Helene Diamantides (now Helene Whitaker) led the way at the same inaugural Dragon's Back event, from Conwy Castle in north Wales to Swansea in the south. An alumni of Mountain Marathons, Whitaker had more than proved her prowess at endurance. In 1987, alongside fellow fell-runner Alison Wright, she broke the world record for running from Everest Base Camp to Kathmandu in Nepal. They did the 188-mile (303 km) mountainous route in three days and 10 hours. With this experience in her back pocket, the Dragon's Back did not phase her at all. She had tested her ability to run for days over mountains many times. And she wasn't even wearing kit designed for her sex. Instead, Whitaker had to seek out the narrowest men's shoes she could find and wear shorts over running tights to cover the flap installed to allow men to urinate. 'In 1992 there was no such thing as adventure racing, it hadn't been invented yet. We were not even running in lycra, mobile phones weren't available', she said.

This new event was about competitors finding their own way, at their own risk. To Whitaker, it was incredibly appealing. Not least because it would be an amazing experience to have traversed Wales along its highest mountain points. Feeling that she would be in with a good chance of success, she signed up as a female team and began to prepare meticulously. No one knew what the race was going to be like. It had never been done before. But Whitaker recced as much of it as she could, bought all the maps and worked out routes in advance. She discovered some of the route went around farmers fields and some footpaths were cut off. In the end her female partner had to drop out because she was unwell. Never missing a beat, Whitaker had accounted for this eventuality and had already asked Martin Stone to be on standby. He stepped up and with Whitaker's intense preparation and research into the route, they went on to win the race. 'I was there to give it a really good chance. I was setting out to do the best I possibly could.' Their first-place position all came down to the final day. She knew they would be at their best in the mountains and slower on the flat. Whitaker anticipated this and planned her strategy around it. They had raced together as a pair before and knew each other's strengths and were able to play to them. In her long experience, women who take part in these extreme events 'do their homework'. They come better prepared than the men and wouldn't even attempt it if they couldn't navigate. 'I've often joked that the best of luck comes to those who are best prepared, but it's not really a joke and I think women become confident going into it with a little bit more preparation.'

...

Though few in number, the small band of early female endurance athletes were 'absolutely crucial' in how women's running has progressed since. These women are the rockstars of the early ultra world, but very little is written about them. Katie Holmes, a runner and historian, has tried to right this wrong by documenting the achievements of the pioneers of endurance running in the UK, including Eleanor Robinson's early ventures. She wanted to learn more about those 'rule breakers' who had not been acknowledged. Others she has come across in her research include Ann Sayer who was born in 1936. 'She's a really interesting example, because she started off rowing, she represented Great Britain, at a time when the sport was in its infancy but then she became interested in walking and in 1977 she and another woman, Dianne Pegg, managed to get into this 100-mile race.'

A geologist who worked for BP, Sayer became fascinated by the Centurions – the feat of walking 100 miles in 24 hours. But with no official long-distance race walks for women in the 1970s when she was training, she also had to battle to get a man's race to accept her entry. Finally in 1977, she was allowed to enter a race in the Netherlands and completed it in 21 hours and 45 minutes. That same year she became the first British Centurion after coming 11th in the Bristol 100 Mile Walk completing it in 20 hours and 37 minutes. In Spring 1979, Sayer set a world record for the longest distance walked in 24 hours (187.7 km) before taking on a 420-mile (676km) three-peak challenge over the three highest mountains in Scotland, England and Wales. She did that in just over seven days, beating the previous record set by a policeman the previous year by 11 hours. It took until 2024 for up-and-coming ultra runner Imogen Boddy to beat her time for the new women's record. The kit, support crew, fuel and training Boddy had at her disposal would have been unrecognisable to Sayer. Holmes refers to Sayer as a 'real groundbreaker', with her consistent pace and power of endurance earning her the nickname of 'Metronome Sayer'. Continuing to participate in a wide range of events, representing Great Britain and at one point getting the world record for the 840-mile (1,352km) Land's End to John O'Groats Walk, she never sought attention for her achievements but her determination opened up long-distance races to other women.

...

These female ultra trail pioneers were not a UK-specific phenomenon. In the US, a small group of female ultrarunners were also making their mark in the 1980s. Sally Edwards who competed in the trials for the first Olympic marathon had just a few years earlier in 1980 won the Western States 100-mile women's race, beating her nearest rival by just two minutes. Edwards moved into multi-sport events and later became known for supporting women to compete in triathlons by coming last 125 times so that no one had to worry about being the final finisher. Another leader of the sport, Ann Trason, has been described as the most successful female ultra runner of all time. At school she had run with the boys in cross country races and had been involved in club athletics. In her first 50-mile race, she not only won, she set a course record. Her driving force for that run – at the tender age of 25 – was to prove to her idol Edwards, who was also in the race, that she had what it took. After that initial heady success, Trason admits it did take her some time to find her feet in ultra running due to making 'every mistake under the sun' including overtraining and not eating or drinking enough.

A major barrier to reaching her potential was that the resources at her disposal were all based on men. Training plans, nutrition, kit. Not one bit of it had been designed for the female body and she soon realised she needed to adapt. A natural problem solver, this was just one more issue to fix. At first she ran way too much, copying Chuck Jones, an ultra runner who had been doing 180 miles a week in training. 'I thought that's what you had to do but my body can't handle that kind of mileage. I ended up with my knees really injured and it took me two failures at Western States to learn from all of the dumb things I was doing.' Trason realised she would need to find her own way. She sat down and wrote out all the things that had gone wrong and a strategy for what to do differently. She loved the camaraderie of her ultra-running friends, she relished the challenge and the problem solving and so she persisted. Trason built in more rest days and easy runs into her weekly schedule. She taught herself to be in the present, checking in with her body to stay ahead of problems, whether it was needing more food or water, or dealing with a blister. She slowly learned what foods were easiest on her stomach when running 100 miles.

She ignored what the men were doing and went on to have a phenomenal ultra running career breaking record after record including winning Western States 100-mile race 14 times. The first time she won in 1989, she also became the first woman to come in the top ten. By 1994 she had won the women's race six years in a row, achieved a course record that would stand for 18 years and was second place overall. In all, she broke 20 world records. In the 1990s, for two years in a row, she did the double of winning Western States just 12 days after winning the 56-mile Comrades race in South Africa, a hilly and fast road race known for being brutal on the feet. 'It is how you deal with things when they are hard that really shows your character. The worst thing you can do is have a failure and not learn,' she said. Trason seemed to be able to run ultra after ultra with no adverse impact. If anything, she got stronger with each one.

In 1994, she did something still viewed as an impossible feat at the Leadville 100 – also known as the Race Across the Sky – held in the Rocky Mountains. That year saw the best runners of the Tarahumara, a tribe native to Mexico's Copper Canyon with stunning endurance running ability, pitted against the ultra elite of the day. With steely determination, Trason came second overall, far ahead of five of the six Tarahumara runners setting a female course record that remains an hour faster than any woman has run it since. A fairly shy Trason never really got the recognition she deserved for her achievement against the Tarahumara runners. Hers was not the story the media focused on. The tale came to prominence more than 15 years later in 2009 when journalist Christopher MacDougall told the tale of the Tarahumara in his New York Times bestseller Born to Run. Here was a tribe that could run incredibly fast over long distances without the injuries that plagued runners with all the latest shoe technology. Such was the book's popularity, it started a trend for barefoot or minimalist running shoes. In 2006, MacDougall travelled with the ultra runner

Scott Jurek to Mexico to learn from and compete in a race with the Tarahumara. The book, told largely from a male perspective, was an overnight success and brought tales of ultra running to the masses. And while it did outline Ann Trason's stunning Leadville run in 1994, this was structured amongst a narrative of political rows between promoters and coaches who had courted the publicity surrounding the race. Trason is depicted as an exceptionally talented runner, but also as a stubborn outsider, taunting the tribe by attempting to defeat them. It recounts her interview at the end of the race where she said 'sometimes it takes a woman to bring out the best in a man'. Despite being one of the most popular running books ever written, few would remember Ann Trason's role or her record-beating run from reading it. Women, it seems, are so often secondary characters.

5.
VICARIOUS ABSENCE

A network of cables lay abandoned on the desolate studio floor. Discarded coffee cups sat unattended on the empty worktops, drained of their final dregs. The electric buzz which had filled the room just three hours earlier was reduced to a lonely hum. A huddle of lone figures sat in isolation eagerly awaiting the arrival of Australian Lucy Bartholomew. Outside, the awe-inspiring mountains were cloaked in darkness, but the town of Chamonix in the French Alps was still a hub of activity. Spectators gathered outside restaurants, drinking red wine, lapping up the charged atmosphere of the most competitive trail race in the world. Inside the commentary booth, it was a different story. Throughout the first 22 hours of the 100-mile (160km) Ultra-Trail du Mont-Blanc (UTMB) race a throng of broadcasters filled the studio commentating in seven languages. The live coverage beamed to YouTube as hundreds of thousands of viewers tuned in to see the race unfold. As a Chinese runner, Fuzhao Xiang, crossed the finish line in fourth place floating the national flag above her head, the TV crews began to pack up their gear. By the time fifth female Maite Maiora Elizondo finished her race 35 minutes later, the studio was bare. All except English-language commentator Corrine Malcolm and her male co-presenters. She was committed to seeing in the top 10 women. Disheartened by the departure of her media counterparts, Malcolm remained resolute that she would be the voice of the elite women's field. 'We were the only channel that stayed on with live commentary to bring in the fifth through to the tenth in the women's UTMB field. The entire studio was empty. It felt disrespectful. We had made a commitment that if we're going to cover the men's top 10, we're going to cover the women's top 10. That shouldn't be going above and beyond, that should be the minimum standard.' Malcolm's experience was not unique. It certainly wasn't the first time she had been left in this position. In mixed races, men's results by default were highlighted first with women's performances viewed as an added bonus. A desirable rather than an essential. And pushing back against this blatant sexism ultimately cost Malcolm her job. But her fight didn't stop there.

...

The depressing truth is that while the number of women taking part in competitive events has grown, these races continue to be viewed through the male lens. It's no wonder that pregnancy deferral, sanitary products and women's safety are not on the radar of many race directors and commentators (see more in Chapter 18). Many sports women don't get equal prize money or salaries, they often attract lower sponsorship revenue, and they aren't allowed to compete in the same distances as men. Everything from bicycle saddles to running tees, through to hydration vests, are developed in an industry where the attitude of 'shrink it and pink it' for women still prevails. Kit is designed for men and then made smaller for women. Sadly, this isn't just in the world of professional sport. It starts in the school playground where break time is dominated by boy's games driving the stereotype that sport is a man's world where women do not belong. Since 1984, Women in Sport, a UK not-for-profit organisation, has been driving change to tackle gender inequality in sport. But change has been glacial. The charity's 2023 report concluded: 'The underlying narrative implies that girls are not as competitive; that sport is not important for girls; that they will never be as good at it compared to boys.' While some may foolishly believe we live in a feminist utopia, sexism in sport is not from a bygone era. Women feel it every day whether it's being sidelined in coverage, being forced to wear sexualised sportswear or having their abilities questioned. Fell runner Sabrina Verjee (see Chapter 14) vividly recalls how her male teammates refused to let her navigate on multi-day adventure races even when she was coping with sleep deprivation better than them. 'I started to grow tired of the déjà-vu experience of racing with three men who treated me as though I was there to be seen but not to speak my mind. Despite me having far more experience than the men inviting me to race with them, their idea of my contribution to the team was simply to fulfil the female requirement. I enjoy logistics and map reading but it was clear the guys had no interest in letting a woman do these things.'

The dismissal of women's abilities is repeated throughout society, not least in the underlying narrative portrayed by a sports media which fails to give equal coverage to both sexes. Despite some progress, an enormous gender gap remains. Coverage of women's sports accounts for less than a seventh of UK sports on mainstream TV channels, a bleak reminder that gender imbalances persist in the commercial world. This has led to mistakes in media coverage as reporters assume men are always faster. They don't have a nuanced insight into women's achievements. When an ultra runner, Damian Hall, won the 2023 Spine Race, breaking the male course record, much of the media reported it as an overall record. They did not think to check whether the outright record was held by a woman or a man. At the time it was held by Jasmin Paris and Hall's win was still 90 minutes behind. This underestimation of women creates a social and cultural environment whereby female accomplishments are reduced to the serendipity of luck, easy conditions, or male heroics. When Paris became the first female to ever complete the Barkley Marathons (see Chapter 20) she was once more met with worldwide headlines. In one report on the website Run247, a male journalist implied Paris had only finished because she was helped by a man. The headline read 'One of the great sporting gestures: How Jared helped Jasmin to Barkley Marathons immortality'. Meanwhile, days after Paris' victory, the podcast Bad Boy Running recorded an episode discussing whether the Barkley had got easier. Similarly, when adventurer Jamie Aarons traversed the 282 Scottish Munros setting an outright record of 31 days (see Chapter 13) one commentator claimed she only beat the time set by Donnie Campbell because she had better weather. Meanwhile, much of the media seemed aghast that a middle-aged social worker could be quicker than a former marine. Lynne Cox, an American, was deemed to have beginner's luck when she became the fastest person to swim the English Channel (see Chapter 11).

Hundreds of years after the first women proved their mettle in the sport of pedestrianism, female achievement is still not given equal weight to men's. It is not deemed as significant, as worthy or as believable. Women's accomplishments continue to fight for equal coverage, equal prize money and equal sponsorship in sport. Women in sport are all too often invisible. A comparative study of women's sports coverage in the UK national press before and after the 2012 Olympic Games found no evidence of an Olympic 'legacy' in increased coverage. Corrine Malcolm's experience in the French Alps illustrates that more than a decade later, sports newsrooms are still routinely failing to redress this balance. The ultra-endurance field is just as guilty as the rest of sports for ignoring women. As the only female reporter on the UTMB English channel commentary team, Malcolm is keenly aware how female authorship in sports journalism is marginalised. Across the globe around 90 per cent of sports reporters are male, according to the International Sports Press Survey. While this study was conducted in 2011 more recent studies report similar findings in the USA and UK. In 2021, the National Council for the

Training of Journalists reported that only seven per cent of those registering for accredited sports journalism courses in the UK were women. This gender bias leads to a sports ecosystem where reporters neglect, or even forget, the accomplishments of women, when they are lionising male winners.

...

While Malcolm was on the sole commentary team waiting to see in the top 10 females at UTMB, the male winner Jim Walmsley was asked on the finish line how it felt to become the first American to win the race. He swiftly corrected the journalist that he was the 'first US man' to do so. 'It just feels like I get to join the strong US women contingent. They've done it again and again here and I'm just happy to stand on their shoulders,' he said. Malewashing of female achievements is something British Grand Slam tennis champion Andy Murray has been calling out for years. At a Wimbledon press junket in 2017 the former world number one corrected a journalist after being asked about Sam Querrey 'becoming the first American to reach a Grand Slam semi-final since 2009'. Murray interjected with 'male player' twice, as the reporter had overlooked Serena and Venus Williams, Madison Keys and Coco Vandeweghe, who had all qualified for Grand Slam finals since 2009. At the unveiling of a 2023 poster celebrating past and present Wimbledon greats, Murray again highlighted the lack of prominence given to female players, who had been pushed to the background of the artwork. As these examples demonstrate there is a systematic lack of visibility of elite women in sport. Women are not seen. They are also not heard.

As a board member of the Pro Trail Runners Association, an athlete-owned organisation dedicated to equality, sustainability and fair play, Malcolm frequently works with races to try to broaden their commentary. She believes world-class events like UTMB have a responsibility to change the status quo and usher in positive change.

Pushing from the inside was Malcolm's mantra and until December 2023 UTMB kept inviting her back to voice her opinion on how to improve commentary. Working as a freelancer for the organisation for four years she was also not afraid to be critical on air. At the 2023 race, she collected data on the amount and quality of airtime given to the elite women's and men's field. Something which she believes made the race organisation twitchy. Attending a meeting at the end of 2023 to discuss commentary of Chiangmai Thailand, part of the UTMB World Series, Malcolm claims she was ambushed. 'I was told I had been too critical of the organisation and so they couldn't work with me,' she said. 'But I think you should be allowed to love something passionately and be critical of it because you want it to be better. I am not a spokesperson for UTMB. I am not employed by them. I take my time on the mic seriously but it's also my responsibility to support and protect and represent athletes.'

UTMB did not want to comment on Malcolm's claims, but pointed to the work it is doing to increase female participation.

Holding out for a public apology, Malcolm has distanced herself from UTMB and embraced working on an all-female commentary team for the 60k Black Canyon race in Arizona, USA. She's also taken proactive steps to make visible change. In her role at the Pro Trail Runners Association, she co-founded the HERE FOR THE WOMEN'S RACE T-shirt campaign to call out the poor coverage of the female competitors in live trail running productions. The initiative uses the funds from tee sales to support the Women's Trailrunning Fund, bombastically pegged as the 'WTF' scheme. The fund issues grants to applicants seeking to increase the visibility of untold and overlooked female stories in trail and ultra running. Malcolm and her colleagues are seeking to change the status quo so the next generation of girls feel seen. Despite much resistance Malcolm continues to open up conversation on gender parity in the sport she loves. As a professional ultra runner herself she is acutely aware of the disparities in the sport and fiercely defends equitable treatment. Sponsored by Adidas

Terrex, the Seattle-based athlete discusses pay with her teammates, an activity encouraged by the brand. 'They have gender-matched it pretty darn well and told us we can talk about it because they are confident that we are not going to find our male counterparts are being paid more. But I don't think that is the same brand-to-brand. Male athletes are still getting better contracts, particularly at the higher level of the sport.' The vast majority of elite male sportsmen are paid a higher percentage than female elites achieving the same results for the exact same sponsors. The Forbes 2024 highest-paid athletes list featured no women.

...

The dearth of parity is alarming. There is a gender pay gap. There is a gender coverage gap. There is a gender expectation gap. Yet participation requires vicarious confidence. When women see people like themselves engaging in ultra endurance they perceive it as a space for them. When women are largely absent or sidelined by their elite male counterparts, these events are deemed too hard, too masculine, too unfitting for a female. The vicarious absence perpetuates a vicious cycle where many women feel endurance is not an appropriate or welcoming activity, so fewer take part, meaning numbers are thin on the ground. The starting line in ultra sport becomes invisible to women making it impossible to decipher what they are truly capable of.

6.
INVISIBLE STARTING LINE

Stepping onto the ice for the first time the little girl hesitated. Her blades touched the merciless surface which glistened under the harsh lighting of the Dublin ice rink. The cool air prickled her skin as she anxiously surveyed the dome. Her eyes darted across to a group of unruly teenagers scattered across the ice twisting into contorted poses as they grappled with the slippery terrain. Suddenly, a boy with flailing arms slid past her uncontrollably, smashing into the wall with a painful thud. She momentarily considered retreating to the safety of the stands before pushing the intrusive thought away. It was now or never. Tucking her neat dark locks behind her ears Jackie Kabler took a deep breath and pushed her right foot forward. She had no idea what would happen. The girl who couldn't hit a ball in hockey, didn't know how to dive in swimming and had never been picked for a school sports team, expected to land unceremoniously on her backside. She braced herself for impact. This was going to be embarrassing. But as she lifted her left leg behind her something unexpected happened. Kabler smiled. The beam spread across her face until it felt like the corners of her mouth would touch her eyebrows. A flash of crisp air washed over her cheeks as her feet found their way, effortlessly, across the rink. She glided graciously, picking up speed as she whizzed past her classmates. In the centre of the arena stood Kabler's PE teacher, mouth wide open, eyes popping out of her head. Rubbing them in disbelief she muttered: 'I think you've found your sport'. 'Thanks Miss,' replied Kabler timidly, amazed at the positive comment from her teacher. It was the nicest thing Miss had ever said to her. 'Maybe I'm not useless at sport after all,' she thought to herself. The next hour felt like a dream, as the teenage Kabler flew around the ice rink like a rocket. She was a natural. Then just like that it was over. The children piled back onto the school bus and Kabler never went ice skating again. Her crowning glory in sport was over before she had even started. It was thirty years before she felt the athlete's high again.

Attending secondary school in Sligo, Ireland, it soon became apparent to 12-year-old Kabler that there were two types of girls. Sporty girls and academic girls. While the boys were encouraged to be all-rounders, the girls were placed in opposing categories. 'I missed out on so many years of sport. I was always top of my class on the academic side, but I was a completely non-sporty person, and that ingrained itself in my head. I thought I just wasn't good at any sport. If I hadn't been good at reading or maths, I would have been given more support but because it was sport, nobody cared or bothered. I wasn't encouraged in any way, and I didn't encourage myself.' While Kabler was confident in her academic abilities it didn't filter through to her sporting capabilities until much later in life. Sport was something the boys did at the weekend, whilst she went shopping with her girlfriends. This extended into adulthood as her aversion to sport took hold, creating an unfavourable lifestyle. As her career in broadcast journalism soared, her health deteriorated. She travelled the world reporting news for the British breakfast TV show GMTV, staying in hotels, eating unhealthily and avoiding breaking into a sweat. As a slim size 10 youngster she had only viewed exercise as a means to stay thin, something which came naturally to her without the need for physical activity. But it wouldn't last forever.

Once she hit her thirties things began to change and the unhealthy lifestyle became more apparent. In a bid to lose weight she began following exercise videos before deciding to take up running. Soon it wasn't about losing weight, it was about feeling fit, healthy and happy. By age 40 she was a regular solo runner, running 10km three times a week. Growing in confidence each year, by her fifties she was ready to push herself further. She ventured into the world of ultra running, taking on 24-hour events and setting personal challenges to run 10 half marathons for 10 days, and three marathons for three days. By the age of 58, she had run 70 miles continuously, spurred on by vicarious role models like Jasmin Paris. And while Kabler was childfree, she had a busy career working three days a week for shopping channel QVC whilst writing crime novels four days a week. These days there are no barriers preventing Kabler from running. She does not doubt that sport is for her. 'I have realised that I can do it. And I don't see why I can't keep on running further. I'd like to run 100 miles. I've also learned that I can fit it in. I just have to prioritise it. Every week I look at my diary, and all my runs, and that's the first thing I put in my diary and then socialising and everything else afterwards.' This newfound confidence is bittersweet for Kabler. She loves being able to push further as she ages but can't shrug off the feeling she lost years of opportunity. That school and society stole her sporting self-belief and stifled her potential. That aside from one blissful afternoon on the ice, no-one ever believed she was good at sport. And whilst she may have been a teenager in the 1980s, sadly, her experience is not confined to the past.

Society is shifting, but the changes are far less radical, and the pace is far more glacial, than little Kabler could have hoped for. Girls in the UK may be given one pitch to play football at break time, but the remaining pitches are still dominated by boys. When girls do participate in sport the bar is set much lower. Cross-country races have shorter distances, and this permeates into the women's races. 'Women and girls are conditioned from an early age to underestimate their abilities, to be princesses rather than superheroes,' says Maud

Hodson, founder of the Run Equal campaign, set up to equalise the distance in UK cross country. 'Differences in race distances – which start in the junior age groups – are part of this insidious, ingrained sexism. Athletics should empower girls and women, not keep them in their place. Just as importantly, it shouldn't give boys the idea that their event is more challenging or more important.'

Women's abilities are underestimated in the Olympics even now. Distances in many sports such as swimming and canoe-kayaking continue to be longer for men than women, for no physiological reason. Tennis is a fine example of the ongoing, unsubstantiated debate surrounding women and endurance. More than 145 years after the Wimbledon tennis tournament was launched, men and women still play a different number of sets. This disparity is retained in the Grand Slams of the Australian Open, the French Open and the US Open, where men play the best of five, and women best of three sets. There is no scientific evidence for this protocol, and it actually goes against precedent. From 1891 to 1901 women played best of five sets in the US National Championships, the predecessor of the US Open. There was also another brief stint between 1984 and 1998 when women were permitted to play five sets in the finals of the Women's Tennis Association championships, following Billie Jean King's 1973 defeat of Bobby Riggs in the legendary Battle of the Sexes. This internationally televised exhibition match saw King beat Riggs in three straight sets in response to his taunting of female tennis players. Outside of Grand Slam competition women continue to play five-set matches but when it comes to the centre court the concept that women are not as physically capable as men, over a longer period of time, is reinforced.

This litany of messages spreading the view that women are not as physically capable as men filters down into school with numerous studies demonstrating that limited expectations are placed on girls. While 70 per cent of boys aged seven to 11 take part in team sport, just 49 per cent of girls do the same, according to a revealing UK Women in Sport study. Kabler was never taught how to hit a ball with a tennis racquet or given the skills to dive correctly into the school pool, so assumed she was not sporty. Four decades later and the picture remains the same. Girls in school are still not supported adequately to develop fundamental movement skills to participate and enjoy sport, leading them to believe they have a lack of natural ability and will therefore never be good enough, says the aforementioned 2023 report. Inquiries by the America Women's Sport Foundation came to similar conclusions. A national US study of parents found they tended to place a higher value on sport for their sons than their daughters. In the US, girls enter sports later, participate in fewer numbers, and exit earlier than boys. Between the ages of six to 10, girls' involvement in sport lags behind boys by 10 percentage points. And yet there is still a greater focus on investing in male sport, with boys receiving more than 1.13 million more sports opportunities at US high school than girls.

The lower expectation placed on female physical prowess feeds into the notion that women do not have a natural aptitude for sport. Whilst the boys were encouraged to be academic and sporty at Kabler's school, the girls were strictly segregated into one category or another. Not both. So, it comes as no surprise that by the early teenage years sport becomes associated with feelings of 'I'm not good enough'. Rather than an opportunity for development and enjoyment, sport in adolescence is viewed by girls as an opportunity to fail. Women in Sport's investigation into puberty and sport found 35 per cent of girls did not participate due to a lack of confidence. The long-term consequences of this can be difficult to reverse. As a charity dedicated to transforming sport for the benefit of every woman and girl in the UK, Women in Sport collates multiple data sets each year. Its findings indicate that by the age of 17, only 28 per cent of girls describe themselves as sporty compared to 58 per cent of boys. This gap continues into adulthood with women in every age group less active than men. Stephanie Hilborne, CEO of Women in Sport, says: 'Girls are being held back by gender stereotyping. Rather than being encouraged to achieve whatever they set their mind to, they're surrounded by messages telling them they're fragile, weak and don't like competition. We know that sport can teach pivotal life skills like resilience, courage and self-belief, but far too many girls are missing out as they're being pigeonholed into what society expects of them.'

Traditional gender role beliefs retain a strong grip on young women with some teenage girls deeming sport an unfeminine and unattractive activity. This is compounded later in life during the menopause, which symbolises a loss of femininity for some women. This perceived deficit increases the fear of judgement in sporting environments, because women feel more vulnerable and at risk of being perceived as masculine. The belief that to be sporty, is to be defeminised, feeds into the gender stereotype that sport is not for females which can lead to exclusion. Women in Sport revealed that 57 per cent of parents of girls said their daughter had felt excluded from sport and 26 per cent of girls had heard that sport 'wasn't for them', echoing Kabler's high school experience all those years ago. For these young women the thought of entering an ultra-endurance event for fun may be beyond consideration. The starting line is not visible to them. It is an activity reserved for world-class professional female runners and not within the realm of possibility for the everyday woman. While men may also be intimidated by the distances involved in ultra running, cycling and swimming, the lack of self-belief is far more prevalent in women. There is both anecdotal and empirical evidence for this. 'I do notice less belief in my female athletes and less confidence,' says British ultra-running coach Damian Hall, who coaches around 40 athletes a year. Numerous scientific studies have demonstrated a confidence gap between the sexes, with men often being over-confident and women sometimes under-confident in their skills and performance.

Confidence is undoubtedly a barrier for many women but those who do possess the self-belief to take on an ultra-distance event have an even greater hurdle to overcome. Time. Women have five hours less leisure time than men per week and it's only getting worse, according to the UK National Office for Statistics. Globally, men are now taking a lot more time each week for leisure whilst women are taking much less. More women are in employment, meaning they have less time to spend on themselves, because when they are not working, they prioritise family commitments. In America, working men have more leisure time than working women, according to data from the Bureau of Labor Statistics. Across every age group in Australia, men have on average four more hours of leisure time than women, as recorded in the last census. Women take on a greater burden of housework, childcare and the caring of relatives and hold the belief that signing up for anything over an extended period of time would be 'selfish', according to the startling findings of a report by Women in Sport, Barriers to Sports Participation for Women and Girls. Although men also have to find time to train for ultra-endurance events, they have more time readily available.

Women have greater difficulty with 'negotiation-efficacy' and being able to fit training around work and family. This was discovered by researchers at the University of West Scotland who set out to understand the enablers and barriers experienced by women and men participating in ultra marathons. Although time was a barrier for both sexes, the research concluded that females may be less confident in negotiating training time. There was also an inherent 'reduced sense of entitlement to leisure' existing in women with caring responsibilities. Women cited delaying taking up running due to having young children, whereas male runners did not. More telling was that the number of men with dependents taking part in ultra races was significantly higher than women with dependents. Far more fathers were racing than mothers. 'Restrictive gender roles persist and these may influence the negotiating-efficacy of female ultra runners more than males, thereby potentially reducing availability of female training time,' the researchers concluded. Their study also noted that women still struggle to negotiate leisure and sport access in an environment where 'discourses of 'good motherhood' continue to denote women as the primary caregivers'. The existence of 'mum guilt', a term often used playfully by a mother to rationalise missing a training run or not signing up for a race, has huge consequences for participation. Data from Women in Sport demonstrates that mothers often put their needs behind everyone else, which makes prioritising physical activity difficult.

This gender gap is especially prevalent in the field of endurance sport, which requires extended hours of training. Subsequently, female participation rates remain low. The amazing achievements of Jasmin Paris (Chapter 1) and Eleanor Robinson (Chapter 4) may give the impression that women are shaking off expectations, breaking boundaries and exploring their full potential en masse, but these athletes remain the exception. Whilst 10km, half marathon and marathon races often have a relatively equal split of women and men, the distribution is far starker at ultra distances. Participation rates clearly demonstrate that the longer the distance, the lower the female participation. Gender parity is strongest in parkrun, an informal 5km run, jog, or walk, every Saturday in parks across the world. More than 1.2 million people in the UK, Ireland, Australia and South Africa registered for parkrun in 2019, over half of whom were female. In the UK, females accounted for 53 per cent, rising to 57 per cent in Ireland and South Africa. Numbers in half marathon distance are also growing, with a Swiss study finding women were 12.3 times more likely to run a half, than a full marathon. But even at marathon distance female participation is relatively healthy. The largest recreational marathon study in history, by RunnerClick, found the global average for female participation was 35 per cent. The results were based on 3.5 million marathon records involving 238 nationalities. American women had the best participant rate of 45.7 per cent followed by Canadians at 41 per cent. The biggest road marathons in the world, the Abbott World Marathon Majors, are attracting females in large numbers. The Chicago Marathon has close to a 50:50 split between women and men, whilst the TCS London Marathon boasts 42 per cent female participation.

Within ultra running these figures take a dramatic nosedive. DUV, the world's largest ultra-marathon database, has logged more than four million performances across 96,000 global races in 200 countries on all continents. Out of the two million ultra runners listed in the directory, 78 per cent are men and just 22 per cent women. Examine each of these countries in detail and it is clear that, globally, men are dominating numbers on the start line. Other datasets are congruous. The most comprehensive study of ultra running, which explored trends between 1997 and 2020, found participation in the sport had increased by 1,676 per cent during that time. There have never been more ultra runners. And while female participation has risen, the Run Repeat research based on 5,010,730 results from 15,451 ultra-running events, found that only 23 per cent of participants were female. Women also have fewer years of running experience and do fewer ultra races than men. Data analysis of 24-hour ultra marathons paints a similar picture, with women accounting for just 19 per cent of the field. In the most competitive races such as UTMB 170km, these rates drop to 12 per cent. The latest figures from a race entry provider, Let's Do This, reveal that since the pandemic women's participation in UK running events has declined by 10 per cent across all distances. Female participation remains lowest in ultras, with 30 per cent of UK ultra runners being female compared to more than half of 5km runners. The figures are even starker in ultra triathlons and cycling. Although studies have shown a fifth of all competitors in 161km ultra marathons are women, this drops to just a tenth in ultra triathlons. Whilst women have won a number of ultra cycling events outright, their appearance on the starting line is still few and far between, usually making up around 11 per cent of finishers. From 1982 to 2011 only 89 women competed in the 5000km Race Across America, 14 per cent of the field. Extreme swimming fares slightly better but is still tipped towards men. Between 1875 and 2013, 1,817 solo swimmers successfully crossed the English Channel, with almost a third being women.

...

Social circumstances unnecessarily hinder female recreational athletes the longer the distance. Women are restricted from exploring their full potential with the status quo determining that ultra endurance is 'unhealthy and harmful' to women's anatomy, according to a study in the International Journal of Environmental Research and Public Health in 2022. A consortium of European sports scientists examined the sex differences in racing history from 10km to ultra marathon and overtly recognised the 'antiquated biases from the 1960s still linger'. The authors concluded that the difference between male and female performances in ultra-running performance may be more closely related to social constraints and expectations of women rather than the physiological advantages of men. 'If you want to understand why there are fewer women participating in these sports and if you want to understand details about the performance, societal and sociological barriers are far bigger factors than any sort of hypothetical about hormonal, or physiological differences,' said Alex Hutchinson, author of Endure: Mind, Body and the Curiously Elastic Limits of Human Performance.

Women face a multitude of barriers. Lower expectations are placed upon girls at an early age, and access to sport is skewed favourably towards boys. Gender ideology conveys the notion that women are carers and sport is a macho pursuit, which only serves to disenfranchise and exclude women. Men's sport is prioritised in the media (see Chapter 5) making women less visible. Kabler is one of the lucky ones. She found her sport. She found her self-belief. She found the time to pursue endurance. She found the races that created a self of belonging and inclusion. But imagine a society where the ultra starting line was visible to all women from birth. What could they achieve given the space to test their limits? On a level playing field could women match men and ultimately surpass them?

7.
SEX MATTERS

In Chamonix, France, a large crowd peers down the narrow sun-dappled streets waiting for a glimpse of the first woman to complete one of the most competitive extreme running races on the planet. In their thousands, they have gathered at the finish line of the Ultra-Trail du Mont-Blanc (UTMB) – which featured in Chapter 5 on TV reporting – to witness the end stages of the merciless challenge, which sees competitors run more than 100 miles over an elevation of 10,000 metres. They know who is likely to be coming round that corner because there is one female athlete who has dominated this race in recent years. A roar goes up when they finally see a flash of a yellow top. Courtney Dauwalter runs at a steady comfortable pace down the picturesque winding street with a wide grin on her tanned face. Her mirrored sunglasses reflect the mass of excited fans taking pictures and sticking their hands out for a high five as cowbells and air horns sound in the background. The mass of banners and flags held by frenzied crowds corralled behind advertising hoardings on the final stretch is reminiscent of the Tour de France. Dauwalter, a former schoolteacher from Minnesota, runs a smooth, easy but fairly speedy pace in her trademark long baggy shorts and oversized T-shirt. At points she is practically weaving her body through the narrow space to get to the end, the number 1 race bib attached to her front. She is smiling from ear to ear as she runs down the blue painted street on the cusp of achieving an epic record. Arms spread wide as she yells in celebration, she has just circumnavigated the highest mountain in Europe. Dauwalter crossed the finishing line, having led the women's race from the start, in a time of 23 hours, 29 minutes and 14 seconds, a full 40 minutes ahead of the next female competitor.

It is the third time she has won the UTMB in four years – a stunning achievement in itself given the calibre of athlete that the event attracts – but there is another extraordinary facet to her win today. A milestone that will put her in the record books and see her crowned not only as the Queen of Ultrarunning but as a groundbreaker of the sport who is surpassing everything that fans and competitors thought possible. Because this is not Dauwalter's first ultra win this year or even her second. In the space of 10 short weeks, she has become the first person ever – man or woman – to do the triple of Western States, Hardrock and UTMB. These historic mountain races are close together on the calendar, which leaves little time for recovery. To do all three, athletes would need to run more than 300 miles over 25,500 metres of elevation gain. In 2023, Dauwalter not only completed them, she obliterated the competition. First in June she set a new record at the Western States 100, winning it in a time of 15 hours and 29 minutes. The next month she set an overall women's record of 26 hours 14 minutes in the Hardrock 100.

UTMB is one of the most high-profile ultra races (with a whole raft of different qualification events that make up the series) but having first been held in 2003, it is relatively new. By contrast, Western States describes itself as one of the oldest endurance races which began when a team of riders wanted to prove that horses could cover 100 miles in one day. Traversing remote paths originally used by Californian gold miners, it was first officially run in 1977 with three runners finishing, only one under 24 hours. Starting at Olympic Valley in California, it crosses canyons and mountains (and one river) on a trail that for large parts is inaccessible other than for runners, horses and helicopters. Weather conditions are highly unpredictable and can go from freezing to heatwave during a single race. It is not for the fainthearted or the underprepared.

Hardrock 100, is another well-known US race within the ultra community. It began more than three decades ago. Participants cover 102.5 miles following that fairly consistent tradition of ultra races being a tad longer than the name suggests. The looped course, which starts in Colorado and is set clockwise and anticlockwise on alternate years, has been cancelled twice since it began in 1992 because of excess snow. As well as being good at ultra running, participants must also have navigation, survival and wilderness skills. The route goes so high up amongst the Rocky Mountains, it has been known to cause some runners to suffer altitude sickness. Many in the community had thought after these two monumental efforts, flying to Europe to take part in the UTMB would simply be a race too far for Dauwalter. Yet the naysayers had vastly underestimated her ability to drive through discomfort, exhaustion and pain. To keep enduring.

At almost 40-years-old, Dauwalter is among those exalted female runners who have won races outright – beating men into second place on multiple occasions. Since she took the leap and quit teaching biology to make running her full-time career in 2017, she has broken record after record. She had always run and had been a state Nordic skiing champion in her youth. Yet it took a while to be the dominant force in ultra sport that she is now. The first time she attempted 100 miles after slowly building up from marathon to 50km to 50 miles, it did not go well. Sitting at an aid station feeling dejected after dropping out of the Run Rabbit Run in Colorado in 2012, she looked up and began to study those who were running past, continuing their journey despite obviously struggling and clearly in pain. It prompted a dramatic shift in mindset from 'how can I do this, to how can I find a way to keep going?' Fast forward two years and she had begun to win those very races that she thought impossible. Four years on from that failed attempt at the Run Rabbit Run, she was the first woman to cross the finish line. The next year she was first female again, despite her sight almost completely failing on the last 12 miles of the race – a terrifying side effect of the strain she was putting her body through. To get that podium place, she had to be talked through the uneven terrain to the finish line by a volunteer. Her vision had turned white and all she could see was her toes. Keeping going had meant tripping and falling multiple times. When she crossed the finish line, she was bleeding from a cut on the forehead.

Dauwalter's trick whenever she hits a barrier or problem to overcome during a race is to repeat the mantra 'You're fine. This is fine. Everything is fine', to herself. To just keep moving and draw on previous experience to work out what she can try to overcome the hurdle. In the toughest moments she descends into her 'pain cave', a space in her mind that she can envisage chipping away at and growing her capacity to cope. 'I just go to work on making it bigger, which helps to stay mentally tough in those difficult moments – and makes my capacity for suffering bigger,' she has explained. Each time she competes, she uses what she has learnt before. Building on past experience, little by little. Dauwalter does not follow traditional training plans or strict nutrition advice. She simply goes by what feels right. It is her ability to use her brain and body together to endure these extreme challenges that keeps her signing up for the next one. 'I want to keep testing myself'. One of the races Dauwalter has won outright is the Moab 240 in 2017. Following the route of the Colorado river, it is twice as long as UTMB, Western States or Hardrock. She completed the Utah course, which winds through dusty desert paths, slick rock, canyons, and mountains, in 57 hours with barely any sleep, finishing 10 hours ahead of second-place runner, Sean Nakamura.

...

Ultra races are unpredictable, with many factors influencing the outcome beyond just strength and power, which are crucial in shorter races like marathons. It is these factors that led Dauwalter to be among the competitors who argue that for endurance events that cover very long distances, like the Moab 240, women stand more of a chance of an outright win. It is possible for them to beat men into second place. 'When I'm out there racing, I don't care if the runner in front of me is male or female. I'm pretty competitive. Winning is always my goal. I think women can compete against men on the same playing field in ultras.'

Outright wins from runners like Courtney Dauwalter and Jasmin Paris have prompted the question whether women can do better than men if a race is far enough. If women are faster in the long run. One oft-cited analysis by the running shoe testers Run Repeat published in 2022 analysed 15.6 million race results from almost 117,000 races in 127 countries. It found that as the distance increases, pace differences seen between men and women start to lessen. In this incredibly large dataset, women started to outperform men at the 195-mile mark. As we discuss later, there are many nuances in how this data can be interpreted. For instance, the fact that far fewer women take part in ultra events and those that do are likely to be among the most well-prepared and well-trained may skew the graph. And it is only one part of a complex puzzle. (Scientists have cautioned that Run Repeat has never released the full data for interrogation.) But its analysis certainly does suggest there are questions to be asked about whether the gap between the sexes diminishes when it comes to the longest of endurance challenges. The notion that women can do better if a race is simply far enough is an attractive proposition. That if you play the long game your time will come. But before delving deeper into this idea, let's ask why this is so astounding. Why is it that we are so shocked when an ultra runner like Dauwalter comes along and seems to flip everything we think we know on its head?

...

In the early 1990s, two physiology researchers based in California wrote a letter in the scientific journal Nature. They had analysed running records from 200 metres to the marathon, decade by decade, to look at improvements over time. The graphs show that women were improving – getting faster and beating previously held records – at a steeper rate than the men. They mapped a trajectory that suggested the gap between men and women would close because of the 'strikingly different' rate of improvements in women's sport. By 1998, the two graphs could intersect, they hypothesised. Looking back on this from our vantage point decades later we know that this did not happen. When the British runner Paula Radcliffe set the women's marathon record in London in 2003, her time of two hours 15 minutes and 25 seconds was eight minutes behind the male winner, Ethiopia's Gezahegne Abera. That same year at the Berlin marathon, Kenya's Paul Tergat became the first person to break the two-hour five-minute barrier. Radcliffe's record in a mixed-sex race was so stunning she held it for 16 years before it was finally broken by Brigid Kosgei in 2019 with a time of two hours 14 minutes in the Chicago marathon. In recent years, advances in shoe technology have led to records being smashed, with Eliud Kipchoge completing an unofficial marathon in under two hours for the first time in 2019. The Ethiopian-born Tigist Assefa hit the headlines after knocking more than two whole minutes off the women's marathon in 2023 running in £400 Adidas 'single-use' super shoes. She had run her first ever marathon the year before. Yet, despite all the advances in technology, nutrition science, and training, there remains an 11-minute difference between the fastest male and female over 26 miles, equating to roughly 10%. This difference is not just seen at the elite level. One analysis of more than 92,000 marathon finishing times found around a 10% difference between men and women at all levels.

Ultras with their varying distances, rules and terrain are a trickier beast to compare, but if you look up the fastest female and male ultra runners in the world over some of the most competitive races, a difference persists at the very front of the pack. By the time Dauwalter crossed the finish line in Chamonix cheered on by those passionate crowds, the male winner, fellow American Jim Walmsley, had been back almost four hours. At Western States that year, Dauwalter set a new women's record but she was sixth overall – and 50 minutes behind the winner Tom Evans. The French winner of Hardrock crossed the finish line three hours before Dauwalter. It must be said that in the world of ultra challenges, these are not particularly long races. Despite the mountainous alpine terrain at UTMB, it can be run quite fast by those at the front of the pack. None of this diminishes Dauwalter's stunning achievement in knocking down record times. But a race with male winners at the front does fit with everything we know about fundamental biological sex differences in physiology and anatomy between the sexes.

Study after study has shown that by and large before they reach puberty, girls and boys are fairly equal when it comes to athletic performance. After puberty, this changes because of the sex hormones that are unleashed as part of the journey to adulthood. Testosterone is particularly responsible for driving fundamental differences in power, strength and speed between males and females. This hormone largely dictates the average 10 to 30 per cent lower performance by women across athletic disciplines, depending on the event. A detailed review of the evidence on sex differences in sport from the American College of Sports Medicine published in 2023 notes that in 2019 more than 10,000 males ran faster times at the 400-metre distance than the three fastest recorded females that year. Here there is no overlap. You can contrast this with sporting events that rely more on skill than muscle power, such as archery, where sex differences are minimal. That improvement in performance among female athletes in the 1990s spotted by physiologists – who took it to suggest that one day women may catch up – is explained by the fact women were in fact playing catch up. Across rowing, swimming, running, jumping and throwing the rate of performance improvement has been faster in women's events for the simple reason that in the early years of competition women were not allowed to enter. They had spent decades pushing back against all the barriers that prevented them even reaching the start line. Finally, the pool of talent taking part was growing quickly and it was showing up in the data. Despite this, average sex differences where strength, power and or endurance are needed remain sizable when you match females and males of similar age and level of training. What scientists are now starting to consider is whether this is always true at the ultra-endurance level: for races far beyond a marathon distance, which can last for days or even longer. There is evidence that women have more fatigue-resistant muscles, are better at burning fat and adopt more even pacing strategies than men – all of which will be covered in forthcoming chapters. But what impact do these advantages have against the benefits that testosterone confers after male puberty?

Testosterone is present in both sexes in different concentrations. It has a wide range of effects but for adolescent boys is the key driver of growth not just in height or size of muscles but also heart and lung capacity. In sport, the impact of testosterone depends on the skill that is required to excel at any individual discipline. For weightlifting – where there is the biggest difference in performance between males and females – size and power are key. Muscle mass and the power it generates can be twice as large in males than females with the biggest differences seen in the upper body, which also corresponds to differences seen in throwing and sprint swimming events. For sports that require heavy cardiovascular demands, such as running, the difference between men and women can be largely explained by something called maximal oxygen uptake, known by the shorthand of VO2 max. Running enthusiasts love to talk about their VO2 max – a measure now included on most smart watches alongside other features such as distance and pace. It is a calculation of the maximum rate of oxygen the body is able to use during exercise. If you have bigger lungs taking in oxygen from the air, and a bigger heart that can pump the blood around the body helping to deliver that oxygen to your muscles, you will have greater aerobic endurance when putting in the same level of effort. In addition to having a higher VO2 max, males on average have higher haemoglobin levels than females, which means they have more red blood cells carrying oxygen around the body to where it is needed. It is one reason that some athletes train for weeks at high altitude camps. They are hoping to boost the concentration of their red blood cells to better oxygenate their muscles. Some experts have pointed out that VO2 max may be less important in very long races, which tend to be done at a slower overall pace, but it is not completely clear to what extent.

Men also have an advantage when it comes to anaerobic power – that intense energy generated over short periods that does not make use of oxygen but instead uses glucose as an energy source. Anaerobic power can be 15 to 50% greater in men, studies have shown, depending on the muscle group, again with the biggest differences seen in the upper body. There are some circumstances where the higher body fat percentage typically seen in women is an advantage – long-distance cold-water swimming being one of them (see Chapter 11) – but in most sports a greater lean body mass is advantageous. On average by the time men reach adulthood, they are taller and heavier, with longer arms and legs.

All of this comes with a big caveat. Athletic ability is not one-size-fits-all and there is wide variation within the sexes, not just between them. These sex differences between males and females are averages. They do not take into account differences in how people respond to training, how they recover after exercise – which seems pivotal to Dauwalter's achievements – and the social aspects of their upbringing and lives that have shaped them as athletes. Nor does it take into account their opportunity of access to sport. Nick Tiller, a sports scientist at Harbor-UCLA in California, is happy to talk about all the ways in which women may be good at endurance sport, but when it comes to the crunch, he wants to know what the science says. As the author of a book dispelling the myths perpetuated by the health and fitness industry, his approach is to apply critical thinking to understand the truth rather than rely on accepted wisdom. He takes an idea and then puts it to the test. In 2021, Tiller carried out a detailed review to try and answer the very question posed by outright wins such as those by Paris and Dauwalter – whether sex differences in physiology advantage female ultra runners. Reporting in the journal Sports Medicine, he found a complex and mixed picture where women appear to be getting closer to men in races of six hours or more. Many factors put women on the front foot in long races such as how fast their muscles tire and how well their bodies use the food they eat along the way. On the downside, women have less ability to take in oxygen and get it to muscles made of up fibres that are smaller in diameter. This cannot be dismissed, Tiller concludes. He is among those who predict that it is 'unlikely that the fastest females will ever outperform the fastest males' in 24-hour ultra-endurance events such as the UTMB. The power and speed conferred by testosterone remain advantageous, at least on the current evidence on these highly competitive 100-mile races. Some argue that these races are set up to favour the men, as outlined in Chapters 5 and 18. Nonetheless, a key part of Tiller's conclusion is that the evidence should be revisited in the coming years, when hopefully the number of female participants has increased and the researchers have more data. Tiller says: 'I've always been interested in the fact that in ultra-endurance sport, the performance gap between males and females is much smaller than it is in apparently any other sport.'

Tiller wanted to collect some original data on what was happening physiologically. So he went to the UTMB to poke and prod some willing guinea pigs and ended up with a sample of around 70 athletes. Only 10 of the athletes were women so to make it fair, he time-matched them with 10 male athletes who would be running at around the same average speed. This small sample threw up some interesting results. All the runners tested negatively on a range of physiological measures he looked at, which is not necessarily shocking given they had just run more than 100 miles. But in the male athletes who'd had blood tests, lung function tests and ultrasound scans, there seemed to be a more negative impact. It included mild post-race pulmonary oedema – fluid accumulation in the lungs – that he only saw in the men. Perhaps the men weren't physically dominant after all. With such tiny numbers, the study could not state whether differences seen between men and women were significant, but the pattern was seen across a range of measures. The race seemed to have had a much larger impact on physiological processes in the men. 'It points to this conclusion that females might be more physiologically robust, to contest these kinds of races,' Tiller explains. Understanding this, however, requires larger sample sizes. What Tiller and his fellow researchers really need is more women to take up ultra sport so they have a larger pool to draw from. At the moment, the women showing up are those who are not intimidated by taking part in a race where 80 per cent of participants are men.

One consideration is that in an ultra, success may be less about VO2 max and more about the ability to push on through damage and fatigue. Tiller remarks: 'It doesn't seem to matter what race you do, it could be a 100-mile race in the mountains, it could be a completely flat race in the desert, by two-thirds of the way through the race, everyone's walking because their legs are completely shot. Your ability to perform seems to be largely related to how well you can sustain that.' Because much of the science in endurance racing is in its infancy, all that can really be said is that the performance gap is the smallest in ultra, he notes.

...

Sandra Hunter, professor in exercise science at Marquette University in Wisconsin, has spent decades studying sex differences in athletic performance and is the lead author of the 2023 review on this topic from the American College of Sports Medicine. It is a potentially contentious subject as governing bodies around the world grapple with how to make sport both inclusive and fair. It is also not one that yet has all the answers. Hunter says on the current evidence there remains a gap overall in performance between males and females in ultra races like those Dauwalter has proven so adept at. Yet even when an athlete is incredibly talented, what cannot be ignored is that in ultra distances, other factors, such as the weather and whether your stomach is handling your food, take a 'bigger portion of the algorithm for success than physiology', she explains. There are simply more variables where female runners can gain an advantage. 'Courtney Dauwalter lives at 12,000 feet and she's getting enormous benefit from that and she works incredibly hard and that's her life. That's her job so she is going to win, particularly these races where there aren't as many people. She will beat a large proportion of the men but she doesn't beat [all] men in the end. There's always a male who comes out top. It's just stacked against women physiologically,' Hunter says. Yet Jasmin Paris' win at the Montane Winter Spine Race shows that women can triumph over men in some gruelling races.

Ultimately, we know lots about sex differences at shorter distances but far less about how ultra endurance fits into this male-dominated picture. In sport, men have always been the standard by which everything is measured – the benchmark. It is one reason why it stands out so starkly when female runners, cyclists, swimmers and triathletes win races outright; because it's not 'supposed' to happen. When Courtney Dauwalter wins a race outright, it makes headlines. But her most stunning achievement to date was in 2023 when she had success at race after race after race in short succession. It shows her remarkable ability to recover. Which begs several questions. What could women achieve if they had the space to fully test their potential?

What could they achieve if we had a better and real understanding of what the female body could do on its own terms?

8.
MIND THE DATA GAP

In an exercise laboratory at McGill University in Montreal, a 21-year-old woman is frantically cycling on a stationary bike. She is one of two dozen healthy active young women who have been asked to do a 10-km time trial as fast as they can. The other instruction she received before her arrival was to bring her favourite, most comfortable sports bra. Overseeing the experiment is Camilla Illidi, a respiratory physiologist originally from Norway, now funded by a sports company, Lululemon, to carry out research into how sports bras influence the mechanics of breathing. In this part of the study, she's testing a high-impact compression bra. It's the type that really straps you down and can be hard to get in and out of. This is being compared with a low-impact bralette with narrow thin straps and limited support. The experiment control is the favourite super-comfortable bra the participant has brought with them. Illidi wants to learn more about the relationship between breast size, sports bras and respiratory muscle fatigue in female athletes. Despite it being almost 50 years since the first commercially available sports bra went on sale, Illidi may be the first person to look into it in any depth.

Sports science has a long history of discounting women. It is far easier to do an experiment on men and then just assume the results are similar in everyone. Females are deemed to be too complicated and messy because their fluctuating hormone cycles can throw the results out of whack. Hormones produced by the ovaries influence a wide variety of processes in the body including metabolism and cardiovascular function as well as targeting a broad range of tissues including muscle. They fluctuate greatly over the course of a menstrual cycle, during pregnancy and throughout a lifetime – and can also be influenced by external factors such as hormonal contraception. In adult pre-menopausal women, for instance, circulating concentrations of oestrogen can vary five-fold and progesterone more than 50-fold over a given menstrual cycle. A menstrual cycle itself can range in length from around 21 to 35 days. It is more difficult but not insurmountable to take account of this in a study. The differing levels and impacts of hormones on women also explain why taking results from studies in male subjects and extrapolating them to females is not the best idea.

While it is slowly and incrementally becoming more common in exercise and sports physiology to look at sex-based differences within a sample, it is still far from the norm. Illidi knows this all too well. During her PhD at university in London, which she began in 2017, she was advised to stick to male subjects because female participants would add a 'level of complexity' that a student could not handle. She felt she had little choice but to take the advice. After all, she was just starting out. Her studies centred around the interaction between airways, lung tissue, ribcage, and respiratory muscles. She learnt a lot, but found it frustrating. 'I know all about the stabilising function of the diaphragm in men because that is what I looked at, but I don't know how that works in women. I guess the work I am doing now is my revenge.' When Illidi moved to McGill University in Montreal she was told she could study whatever she wanted but she had one burning question. She wanted to know whether breast size makes a difference to breathing efficiency in women. Do women adapt their respiratory mechanics depending on breast size? And does the type or fit of sports bra affect that? Illidi runs and cycles regularly and used to take part in Ironman triathlons. For her it seemed like such an obvious question but no one else had asked it, as far as she could ascertain. The 23 women who have pedalled at various intensities on a bicycle in her lab are helping her find some answers. They all have a normal body mass index and a healthy VO2 max (measurement of oxygen intake during exercise). The only difference between them is their breast size. At the end she lets the women keep the experimental sports bras as a thank you for giving up their time. This has had a considerable impact. One young woman with 36DDD breasts took home the high-impact compression support bra and ran for the first time since her early teens.

It is early days, with Illidi only just starting to write up the first findings but she has presented some of her results at a conference in Calgary. The response was shock: how do we not know this already? There is a very simple answer to this question, she explains. Both in London and in Montreal where she is now, she has worked with male scientists who have been approached by bra companies to investigate what impact a sports bra design might have on breathing – but they declined because 'they didn't want to be that guy'. It would probably also never occur to them that breast size might make a difference because they have never felt the impact of an uncomfortable sports bra. 'I don't really care about sex-based differences, I just wanted to focus on what the variability among women might be.'

The evidence she is starting to gather focuses on respiratory muscle fatigue. Generally speaking, the respiratory system is overbuilt for our needs, Illidi explains. In everyday circumstances your legs or arms get weary before your respiratory muscles get tired. Yet if you're an elite athlete working hard in an event to breathe in enough oxygen and get it to the parts of the body that need it, the body has a decision to make. Your brain wants blood flow, the leg muscles want blood flow and so do the respiratory muscles because they need to keep breathing. It would be life-threatening if they couldn't. So the moment those respiratory muscles start to tire, a feedback loop is sent to the brain to constrict blood flow to the legs to keep the oxygen available for the lungs. It is an incredibly complex system with lots of things happening that can be hard for researchers to unpick. Yet there is some evidence of sex differences here, Illidi explains. If you look at someone doing high-intensity exercise, perhaps 80 to 90% of their maximum effort, in general women appear to be better than men at recruiting what are known as the accessory muscles. Rather than relying on the diaphragm to keep the oxygen flowing, women more quickly engage muscles not typically used in regular breathing. These are the muscles in the chest wall, between the ribs and in the neck and shoulders. The muscles that enable really deep breaths, that the body will make use of when having to work harder at breathing. 'So instead of relying solely on the diaphragm, women start recruiting the sternocleidomastoid, the scalenes, and external intercostals to help out with breathing and they do that earlier at around 70 per cent of their max,' Illidi says. Men do it too, but later on once the diaphragm has already started to fatigue which is a little bit too late. Women are doing it before the fatigue sets in. It is a way for the body to spread the work more evenly when having to breathe really hard. Why women might be able to make quicker use of their accessory muscles is another intriguing part of the puzzle, but it could relate to the ability to adapt quickly during pregnancy. 'At some point we might be so mechanistically restricted when having a baby, that we need to be good at activating these muscles to help us breathe,' says Illidi.

The woman peddling for all she is worth on a bike in the lab is helping unpick what impact breast size has on this respiratory efficiency and also what that does to 'perceived effort'. In short, whether the physiological data coming out of the machines matches what it feels like to the individual doing the exercise. It is all being assessed on the bike rather than treadmill, at least for the initial research, because it takes gravity out of the equation with no weight-bearing on the breasts. After asking the women to cycle for five minutes at a carefully calibrated easy, medium and hard pace, Illidi found no differences between breast size and how participants were breathing. The graphs all lined up with each other. Yet the women with large breasts felt very differently about the exercise; they were more aware of their bra, it felt more restrictive, and they reported feeling more uncomfortable with their breathing. It begged the question, what would happen if they were left to do the exercise at their own pace, rather than a rate set by the researchers. If it felt harder and more uncomfortable to breathe – even when physiologically it is achieving the same goal – how would that affect a woman's approach to the task?

The next time, Illidi asked the participants to do a 10-minute time trial going as fast as they felt they could while wearing the high support, low support and old favourite bra. What she found baffled the respiratory research community. When the women chose their own intensity, those with large breasts were breathing much more to get the same level of oxygen into their system (and carbon dioxide out). They were breathing faster but achieving the same result. On the face of it, it appeared like they were not working as efficiently. Over the half an hour time trial, they seemed to be working harder, taking in litres more air every minute. The researchers had also monitored what was happening with the respiratory muscles and found that the women with smaller breasts were very good at recruiting their accessory muscles, taking some of the strain off the diaphragm but those with larger breasts were dependent on the diaphragm to keep their breathing going. The response was similar to what you see with overweight and obese individuals, she explains. But those in the study all had normal body mass index. One hypothesis is if the women with large breasts are having to lift extra weight every time they expand the rib cage, perhaps it is easier for the body to simply breathe more quickly than recruit different muscles. For Illidi, the ultimate aim is to determine the best sports bra to allow someone to breathe in the most efficient way for their body type as well as ensuring they feel comfortable while exercising. The next step will also be to test what happens in a weight-bearing exercise like running.

...

Comfort, rather than efficiency, has been central to the design of sports bras since their infancy. The first sports bra was invented in 1977 by two women who were sick of exercising in their regular underwired bras, which caused sore breasts and chafed skin and had straps that slipped down. They had hunted high and low for an alternative, but none worked satisfactorily. In the end they created the Jockbra, later recoined as the Jogbra, by sewing two jockstraps together. The technology has undoubtedly come on leaps and bounds since that time, but the focus has been on minimising 'bounce' and this key issue of how a sports bra impacts the ability to breathe has not really been part of the story. Illidi references a study conducted 20 years ago that found no restriction on breathing. Interestingly, her research says differently. Decades on from that first sports bra, she is now taking the first detailed steps to consider whether it is best to have a bra that makes you think you're breathing easier or a bra that actually makes breathing easier. Illidi is hunting down that 'sweet spot' where there is as much support as possible without impairing respiratory mechanics that will cause the lungs to tire more quickly.

Someone like Illidi, working in exercise science and researching only women – looking at the variation between them – is a rarity. In an analysis of more than 5,200 studies published in sport and exercise science research between 2014 and 2020, only six per cent were conducted on only females. While almost two-thirds of the studies contained both male and female participants, the proportions were far from even. Of the 12.5 million participants that had been involved in the research over the six-year period, only a third were female. Researcher Emma Cowley and her colleagues concluded, damningly, that at present most conclusions from sport and exercise science research 'might only be applicable to one sex'. Cowley leads the Invisible Sportswomen international research group, a virtual collaboration of researchers based around the world. Having recently moved to the Technological University of the Shannon in Ireland, Cowley has been interrogating this gap from the start of her career. As a PhD student interested in teenage girls' participation in sport, she found very little evidence on the topic. Then she came across one paper which seemed to explain why. It found that women were 'significantly under-represented' in sports research between 2011 and 2014. Surely things would have improved by now, Cowley thought. So during the pandemic, while working at home she decided to bring the study up to date. Using even more journals and a longer timeframe, she found the exact same problem. The figures were almost identical. The needle had not moved at all. This gap in understanding means that, on a very basic level, female athletes are lacking the information on how to approach training, fuelling, injury recovery and more.

The problem perpetuates all fields of sports science. Ella Smith and colleagues at the Australian Catholic University have done several studies looking at what we know about male and female nutrition needs in sport. They found that less than a quarter of participants testing performance supplements were female. In studies looking at carbohydrate intake, women accounted for just 11 per cent of those taking part. Where females were included, most studies included no or little information on menstrual cycles or used the wrong terminology 'suggesting incomplete understanding and concern for female-specific issues'. These are the studies that underpin guidelines and training plans. Yet we do not actually know what the advice should be for women because the research has not been done. Most recently the same team looked at the evidence for heat adaptation – a training strategy used to improve the performance of athletes about to compete in hot conditions – and found that three-quarters of studies assessed only males. In a recently published review of the 100 essential papers in sports and exercise physiology impressively titled 'Standing on the shoulders of giants', only one included female participants. This is an up-to-date list of papers that every student in the discipline should read. Yet women are essentially missing.

Individual researchers can only do so much if the structures they are working in make it difficult to do high-quality research in women. Cowley and her team dug deeper and looked at who was doing sports science research with female participants. It showed that studies led by women were of better quality when it came to the methods they used, because of factors such as taking into account hormone profiles. Yet women are strikingly under-represented in first and last author positions – the most senior roles in the research team.

On top of this there are very practical cost and time implications to doing a study that includes women, Cowley explains. Let's say a researcher is looking at the effectiveness of different types of high-intensity training in the gym. Men could try one session on a Monday and come back the next week and do the next session on the same day. All the data could easily be collected within three weeks. 'But because we're starting at ground zero for women, because we haven't done the research on the impact of the menstrual cycle, we're having to account for it because we don't know if it has an impact or not,' Cowley says. 'It's essentially foundational research where you're having to account for everything.' So if a woman has a 35-day cycle, that data collection expands from three weeks to somewhere near four months. There will need to be blood analysis to track what the hormones are doing. The PhD students who are typically the ones doing the data collection don't have the budget for that and are working within a system where women's research isn't really funded, according to Cowley: 'There are very real barriers.' One of those barriers is if you repeat a study in women that has been well proven in men it is not considered novel research. 'That does blow my mind because we do have different metabolism and different thermoregulation. When it comes to training protocols or nutrition guidelines it might be the exact same for men and women but we don't know. But the response you get when you ask the question is: "Oh, that's been done".'

One issue that researchers will often cite is that it is harder to recruit women to their studies. When it comes to endurance sport, the pool of female athletes, while growing, is still a fraction of the male competitors. But even within a large sports science department with a large number of female students it can be difficult to recruit, says Lewis James, a nutrition researcher at Loughborough University. He's had many conversations with colleagues about why it can take twice as long to recruit enough female participants for mixed studies. His research focuses on the most effective approach to hydration, and he notes that out of 10 to 12 participants who come forward, only a few are women. There may be a whole host of reasons including where and how people are recruited and how comfortable female participants may be sharing personal information or 'testing' themselves in a study. If someone has never done it and their friends haven't done it, they don't know what is involved. Women may also have more caring responsibilities that means they simply do not have time to take part. 'Is it our fault, is it us as researchers because we don't know how to recruit females?' James asks. 'I think there is a piece of work to be done there.' A good starting point would be to consider the language used to recruit female participants, to provide positive messages about the benefits of taking part. Some researchers have reported taking simple steps in the recruitment materials – even the images used on them – can make a big impact. This is similar to the approach taken by race companies aiming to equalise the gender start line (see Chapter 18).

...

Fast forward five years into the future and Cowley predicts things may have moved on marginally. One particularly striking gap she hopes improves is around perimenopause and postmenopausal women – the very demographic who are often breaking barriers in ultra events (see Chapter 17). 'There does seem to have been a change in recent years, people are talking about it more and I've seen a lot more papers looking at the gender gap in specific areas.' This shift in focus is fundamental if society is to encourage more women into sport and help them achieve their potential once they're there. And some good work is already happening. In 2021, Kirsty Elliot-Sale, head of the Centre of Excellence for Women in Sport at Manchester Metropolitan University in the UK, published a guide with a group of colleagues on best practice for including women when designing studies in sport and exercise science. It covers everything from selection of participants to study design. It is not just about collecting more data. That would be meaningless if done carelessly or without thought. It explains to researchers how to generate 'high-quality' female-specific data. Elliot-Sale's statement is a call to arms for future studies to explore the impact of oestrogen and progesterone on women's athletic performance. Better understanding of this in elite athletes could produce those 'marginal gains' that the male team directors of the (all-male) Tour de France get excited about. For recreational athletes, better understanding of how hormone fluctuations impact women's ability to take part in sport in the first place could help reduce the disproportionate drop-off in girl's participation once puberty arrives (Chapter 6). For those taking on ever greater feats of endurance, knowing how to fuel, train and prevent injury is key, including around their menstrual cycle and after menopause.

Some are working to address this issue, including tackling the crucial questions about whether aspects of female physiology offer an advantage in ultra-endurance events. To have any meaningful impact, we cannot simply add women to existing studies. It will require new ways of thinking and a fresh look through a female lens.

9.
EVOLUTIONARY ADVANTAGE

They were working in a team, a pack, to hunt down the deer that would provide much-needed food for the tribe. They knew the ancient land well, every rocky outcrop, wide open plain and forest trail. The sharp spears topped with flint could be used to dispatch the animal; sometimes a rock could do the job. But first their goal was to wear the deer out. The hunters could run for much longer and sweat to regulate their body temperature; it would die of exhaustion or overheating long before they would. As a team, they had been tracking the deer for several hours. It had been a long hard winter but in the summer months the weather was to their advantage because the animal would tire even more quickly. The group knew where the deer liked to graze and drink water, so that was their starting point. Once they had spotted the hoofprints of a potential prey they ran at a steady speed, sometimes walking, particularly if they needed to pick up the tracks of the animal or regroup. Sometimes they could drive the beast off a cliff or into a river to trap it. Other times they fanned out to surround it and force it to keep going while ensuring it had no way of escape. They used the terrain to their advantage; identifying from its tracks when the animal was tiring. At last, success: after hours the deer was overcome with exhaustion, stumbling and about to collapse.

The hunters moved in for the kill, before strapping the carcass to their spears and carrying the animal on the lengthy journey back to the cave, where they would make good use of all its parts.

If most people were honest, when reading this fictional account of an early human tribe stalking an animal for food, clothing, and shelter needed for survival, they would likely imagine a group of male hunters. Perhaps five or six of them, strong and young, wearing hide with great strapping arms carrying powerful weapons. That is the image conjured in the mind's eye because this is what children have been taught from an early age. It is the story in every book written about prehistoric humans. This tale of men hunting while women had children and foraged for berries and plants has completely permeated popular culture. The prejudicial notion that women, being weaker and burdened by pregnancy and breastfeeding, couldn't travel as far has been widely accepted. It was assumed they wouldn't be expected to perform physically demanding tasks. Yet there is a group of researchers keen to turn this portrayal of our early ancestors on its head. The 'man as hunter' theory of the palaeolithic periods is starting to be reconsidered. Part of the reason for this is our better understanding of female endurance ability.

Developing the ability to hunt has long been viewed as a driving force in human evolution. Our human ancestors crafted tools and techniques to chase, catch and kill large animals, adding a nutrient-rich food source to their diet. They were then able to make use of other parts of the animal for clothing and shelter. The prevailing narrative among those studying the period and in modern cultural representations is that labour was divided according to sex differences. Yet on further scrutiny, the evidence does not necessarily correlate with the theory. In terms of who did the hunting, who made and used the tools, who carried the food home, or dealt with the carcass afterwards, the wear and tear on male and female fossil remains are the same. As are the items found at burial sites. What is now being argued is that the evidence has for too long been viewed through a male lens. Or at least seen through the societal lens of the time. This can be traced to as far back as Charles Darwin, who like many Victorians characterised women as passive and submissive. The stereotypical image of the tribe's men embarking on an epic journey to hunt meat – travelling far from the cave, avoiding predators, and using planning and tactics to overcome their prey – while the women handled domestic chores, is, however, largely associated with a theory published in the 1960s. Man the Hunter was first a conference in 1966 and then a book two years later which brought together the evidence on hunting and its central role in human development. The tasks of early hunter-gatherers were divided by sex. Although some challenged this narrative, arguing that it relied on gender stereotypes and assumed that the patriarchal society of today existed 100,000 years ago, this view has become deeply ingrained. Studies have shown that placing men at the centre of palaeolithic life, whether in the textbooks or images used in museums has become more, rather than less, prevalent over time.

Watch a typical nature documentary on hunting and the image is of a faster, more powerful animal gaining and pouncing on a weak member of the herd. Humans take a different approach. For the most part, palaeolithic hunters are thought to have chased down prey until it was exhausted: it wasn't about being stronger or faster but outlasting. A key evolutionary advantage that humans had was they could keep going while the animals they were chasing could not sustain their speed. Endurance was the key to survival for those who had come down from the trees, evolved to move on two legs and extend the range in which they searched for food. For many decades, it was assumed the physical demands of the hunt would be too much for the females in the group who were dealing with pregnancy, lactation and caring for (and carrying) infants – whereas men, physically superior, were considered to be natural hunters. When a four-legged animal galloping to escape was taken down by a powerful throw of a spear, perhaps a fit young man would indeed have hurled that spear. But again, that assumes speed and power were key to a successful hunt, rather than the ability to keep going steadily over a long distance. With a growing understanding of female biology and what that means for endurance, it seems to make little sense to exclude women from depictions of this activity.

...

Cara Ocobock, a human biologist, is a former powerlifter. Whether in a gym or at the University of Notre Dame in Indiana, USA, where she studies how humans adapt to extreme environments, the one thing certain to frustrate her is a lazy stereotype. There was a period when she was harassed in the gym on an almost daily basis by people telling her to not overdo it with the weights or her breasts would shrink. Or that if she lifted weights that were too heavy she would end up looking like a man. She started to wonder where it all came from. Later in her career when teaching a course on introductory anthropology, a fun class exercise started to throw up odd stereotypes. 'It's this really silly assignment where they have to create an online dating profile for the fossil hominin of their choice, for example if Lucy joined Tinder, what would her dating profile look like.' Lucy in this scenario is one of the earliest fossilised skeletons found in Ethiopia in 1978. She was from a species called Australopithecus and her remains, which are about 40 per cent complete, were dated to 3.2 million years ago. She was just over a metre tall and became famous around the world after her skeleton went on tour. The discovery of her bones in East Africa was the first proof of an early human relative that walked upright (although at this point not travelling long distances) before humans evolved to have larger brains. Walking upright is important because it is an efficient way to get around and would have enabled our ancestors to travel more easily from patch to patch to find the resources they needed.

Another famous ancient female was found almost two decades later in the same region of the world. Ardi was 4.4 million years old and sparked a great deal of debate as her skeleton suggested she walked on two legs but also climbed trees. She did not easily fit into the human origin narrative. These famous fossils both significantly impacted researchers' understanding of evolution and both were female. Yet when Ocobock asked her students – a larger proportion of whom were women – to create the joke dating profile as a way of getting them to engage with the subject, almost every single one of them wrote it from the point of view of a man. 'That's what got me thinking about the ways in which we teach biological anthropology and why there is this male-centred focus within human evolution. It almost always defaults to men.'

Ocobock, with her background in weightlifting and interest in women's roles in sports, had also noticed the gap in the research on physiology and exercise science (see Chapter 8). She started to join the dots. As researchers learn more about some of the physiological advantages women may have in endurance sports, their findings put a new perspective on how our ancestors may have lived and sustained themselves. Alongside her colleague Sarah Lacy, she attempted to cast a fresh pair of eyes over the role females may have played in hunter-gatherer societies. In 2023, the pair set out their thoughts in two detailed papers in American Anthropologist, pointing to a wide range of evidence that may have been overlooked in considering what early female humans were capable of. It all depends on the lens you view this through, they pointed out. Simply looking at what might give the male of the species an advantage – longer limbs, larger heart, larger lungs, greater muscle mass – ignores potential female advantages. Take the pelvis. Women have a wider pelvis to accommodate pregnancy and birth and this was long thought to make them less efficient from a biomechanical point of view. Ocobock and Lacy point out that in the past decade studies have shown that this wider pelvis may not actually have any metabolic cost when walking and running because women can potentially adapt the way they walk and run to account for this. Other work has shown that women – thanks to that wider pelvis – may be more efficient at carrying a load on their hip, such as a baby, toddler or a dead animal and moving quickly while doing so.

Then there are hormones. Oestrogen receptors, it turns out, are incredibly ancient. Scientists believe they evolved 300 million years before the androgen receptors that respond to testosterone. Hormones are most commonly characterised as oestrogen for women and testosterone for men, but this is a great oversimplification. In reality, as noted in Chapter 7 both are present in all humans in different concentrations. Best known for its role in ovulation and menstrual cycles, oestrogen also has an effect on metabolism, bone growth, memory, regulating body temperature, mood, how fat is distributed and stored in the body, and adaptation to endurance. Oestradiol – a form of oestrogen made in the ovaries – has been shown to be important in preventing or mitigating muscle damage after exercise. Ocobock and Lacy noted that scientists have shown that females can better withstand periods of environmental instability such as shortages of food. Then there is the evidence that female muscles are more resistant to fatigue (see Chapter 10). Another hormone, adiponectin, is typically higher in females than in males, boosting fat metabolism while sparing carbohydrates for future use (Chapter 11). It also protects muscle from breakdown.

Despite increasing evidence pointing towards females being particularly well-suited to long endurance activities, science has continually 'pulled women out' of the evolutionary story, Ocobock argues. 'We cannot and should not rely on the blanket assumption that females are physically inferior to males and incapable of taking part in the same variety of activities,' the pair concluded. They did lean heavily on evidence from exercise and sports science in putting forward their thesis, and when it comes to female inclusion this evidence is clearly limited, but this is not just theoretical, they stress. There are numerous examples of females hunting in the current day, including the Agta tribes in the Philippines, Inuit in sub-arctic regions of North America, Tiwi people who live on two islands off the coast of Northern Australia and Ojibwa women who live across the US and Canada.

In fact, Ocobock has hypothesised: what if pregnancy, childbirth, and the demands of raising infants did not actually prevent women from participating in hunting? What if that burden has led, over millennia, to the suite of physiological features that make women good at endurance activities. During the final stages of pregnancy and during breastfeeding women use more energy and need to consume more calories. It is not a modern-day phenomenon that women still have all their other work to do while growing and carrying a baby or while feeding a newborn (and beyond), all day and night. From an evolutionary perspective, females would still have had to complete tasks, including finding food and avoiding predators for the nine months of pregnancy and while breastfeeding. They would still have been caring for other young children even in times when food was limited and the weather harsh. With no contraception, this would have been an endurance event in itself as part of a cycle of life that lasted years. As a result, the female body is highly adaptable to accommodate the additional demands being placed on it (see Chapter 12). Fundamentally it makes perfect sense that females have this capability to endure because the survival of the species depends upon it. What if those adaptations are an advantage from an evolutionary point of view, not the hindrance or trade-off that those first positing how humans organised themselves thousands of years ago decided it was, Ocobock wonders.

These theories – and Ocobock and Lacy are not the only ones putting them forward – are just that. They are hypotheses based on the limited evidence available. Once more studies are done on energy use, biomechanics, muscle fatigue and recovery, across the female lifespan from before, during and after the childbearing years, perhaps the understanding of how evolution ties into women's capability in ultra sport will grow. This data can all be put into the evolutionary models that scientists and anthropologists use to try and make sense of how we once lived. But not everyone agrees, says Ocobock, who received pushback after their theory was published in Scientific American. 'It does lead people to say that what we're doing now is woke revisionist history without ever considering the possibility that the original work was heavily biased.' She received hate mail and even had to file a police report. Yet she says that within those studying early human fossil records there was much positive reaction to the argument they made.

...

Science is of course all about thoughtful debate, with ideas rarely fixed. Within some modern-day hunter-gatherer tribes there is more sex-based division of labour. But the Agta women hunt all the time, Ocobock points out, and there are multiple examples of women being very involved with the hunt right up until the point of kill, in terms of planning, tracking, packing out, carrying everything back. 'If you believe the evidence that males were hunting in the Palaeolithic era, then you have to believe the evidence that females were hunting too. Because it's the exact same evidence, everything that we interpret as a hunting behaviour based on bone wear and injuries that we see in our fossil early modern humans, as well as stone tool use and butchery marks, it's the exact same between females and males.' The fossils tell us women were taking the same risks and doing the same activities. It is feasible that a female in the final month of pregnancy or first couple of months afterwards would be taking it easier but then they have to 'get right back to it'.

It turns the accepted wisdom inside out. Rather than women being passive beneficiaries of 'man the hunter' driving forward evolution, this process could have been led by the female body and its endurance capabilities. In her book Eve: How the Female Body Drove 200 Million Years of Human Evolution, Cat Bohannon, an academic and writer based at Columbia University, also challenges the preconceptions of prehistory. It took her a decade to write her stunningly detailed book, which looks at the genesis of endurance ability, busting myths along the way. A reckoning is starting, she says. The story of what females were doing in that hominin past – those species that were the human-like precursor to modern humans – is changing. 'We're starting to realise that females were playing a much more dominant role both socially and in terms of these things we think of as male such as hunting.' For a long time there was an assumption that females could not possibly have been the ones to drive the evolutionary switch to becoming bipedal – moving around on two legs, not four – because they were apparently too weak to walk. Bohannon was not the only one irritated by this assertion and it has been challenged over the past decade, she explains. 'Bipedalism is actually an endurance story, it's a metabolic story and then suddenly it immediately becomes a female story. It flips the idea on its head.'

By about 4.4 million years ago our primate ancestors were walking on the ground and doing so regularly, Bohannon writes. Ardi, the earliest evidence we have of a bipedal ape in our ancestral family tree was 'somewhere between a chimpanzee and a really furry human'. There is much about her bone structure – despite her spending quite a bit of time in trees – that is similar to females today. It is a popular trope among science writers to say that humans evolved to be runners. Probably starting around the time of Ardi and continuing for millions of years, humans evolved to have lighter bones and muscles built for the long haul rather than just short explosive bursts or swinging effortlessly through trees. Human bodies adapted for stamina. What Bohannon argues is there is a good chance 'that females led the charge' for two reasons. One is the metabolic advantage in making efficient use of fat stores needed for pregnancy and caring for young infants, but the other is that Ardi and her daughters may have had more need to leave the forest and venture into the plains.

Most anthropologists probably agree humans evolved to endure – to outrun or even out jog those nimble deer, bison and other animals that could provide a ready meal – but Ardi was not yet at that point as mainly a plant eater. One theory is that human ancestors started to walk further afield to find more food as climate changes made it scarce. Maybe it was not the male of the species going out to bring home the prize for the female, as has been long postulated. She may have been the one pushing further to sustain not just herself but also her young. Bohannon points out that everyone needs food, but for females there was added pressure because they were growing babies while pregnant and feeding them afterwards. To do this you need to be able to endure – especially if you are also carrying needy children with you. Thinking of it this way around places a whole new light on why humans have the most stamina of all. 'There are arguments against this, but I was thinking what happens when your need is not just your own body,' she says. 'What reserves do you have, what are you kicking into.' There is still a lot we don't know, she is keen to stress, whole expanses of time for which the fossil records are missing. And there is a lot of guesswork when postulating these theories. We don't know what the Ardi's or Lucy's of the world were doing on a day-to-day basis. Bohannon says: 'But we do know that the female body seems uniquely adapted to endurance.'

10.
FATIGUE RESISTANCE

When Lael Wilcox saw bicycle lights coming towards her as she cycled on the dark highway in Bumpass, Virginia, she didn't know what to think. After covering more than 4,000 miles across America over 17 days, sleeping for five-hour stints in a grass field, side of the road or sometimes a motel, she was exhausted and wondered if her mind was now playing tricks. After all, who else would be out here in the middle of nowhere at three in the morning. Fairly new to endurance racing, she had turned up to the start line of the 2016 Trans Am Continental Race across America over a fortnight earlier wearing a grey cotton T-shirt and loose brightly patterned shorts with a pair of running shoes on her feet. She was 'a joke' to the others preparing to begin the epic race. The only woman, she was surrounded by intense men wearing serious kit who looked at her like she was completely mad. But Wilcox was fired up and ready to ride hard. Little did they know she had both ambition and deep inner confidence that she could last the distance.

Over the past nine years she had completed gruelling bicycle adventures at home and overseas with no funding or support. Her tour had taken her through more than 30 countries and 100,000 miles over North America, Europe, the Middle East and Africa. Between trips Wilcox would take on temporary work, waitressing or whatever odd jobs were available, doing double shifts and saving up cash before setting off on another journey. She just loved riding her bike. What started as a means of transport to get around and visit family when she had no money and no car turned into a way to explore the world. Competition was almost an afterthought but why not she told herself. Let's see what it's all about. Her first race was 1,000 miles across Israel, where she was the youngest rider and only woman. While everyone around her was stunned to see her leading the race on the first day, Wilcox was hooked. 'I realised I really loved competing and I loved racing these guys, trying to beat them and strategising how I was going to cover more distance each day.'

Those who had dismissed her on the start line of the Trans Am would soon find out just how much they had underestimated the 29-year-old. By the time Wilcox reached the halfway point between the west and east coast she was in second place. Averaging 233 miles a day, she just kept riding and riding. Over mountain ranges – her preferred terrain – and through flat plains, all in the midst of a brutal heatwave that had burned and peeled off her skin twice. Riders fully support themselves at the Trans Am. There are no crews at checkpoints to provide energy gels, massages and words of encouragement. Wilcox stopped sporadically at gas stations to buy pastries, cereal bars, pizza, and chocolate milk to give her the energy to keep going. Sometimes she slept covered by a thin blanket under the stars, other times treating herself to a bed for a few hours. A fortnight into the race there was only one man ahead of her, in fact just 80 miles in front, and with the end in sight, she decided to cut her sleep in half. Just three hours under the porch of a school. The next night was two and a half hours in a field. Bit by bit she was slowly gaining ground, keeping up her relentless pace.

The night she saw the bicycle lights coming towards her, she had only slept for 40 minutes. When the cyclist reached Wilcox, he said nothing, turned around and cycled next to her silently staring at the road ahead. She didn't recognise him at first and wondered if he was a fan of the race. Then she realised he was also dirty, bedraggled and exhausted. Noticing the tell-tale bags on his bike, she asked his name. Steffen, he replied. It suddenly clicked, this was the lead racer she had been chasing since they left Oregon. Steffen Streich, a German ultra-endurance cyclist who the previous year had won the Trans Africa Bicycle Race. He'd also just woken from a short rest but in a sleep-deprived haze set off in the wrong direction. With 130 miles left to go, Wilcox knew this was her only chance and raced off as hard as she could with Streich in hot pursuit. She pedalled away and he caught her, so she pedalled harder and lost him again. Wilcox took a wrong turn at a fork in the road and he shouted at her to go left. Riding together once more, he said 'let's talk' and proposed they finish together. This was not a choice Wilcox was willing to consider. After all this time and effort, a race to the finish was a tantalising option that she did not want to give up. Every time she tells this part, her eyes light up and a huge grin spreads across her face. What happened next gives us some clues about one of the physiological advantages female ultra athletes may have at their disposal.

'This is the best bit, we actually get to race to the end,' she told him. 'After all those hours out there on your own suffering, this is what makes the sport so exciting.' Once more she pedalled as hard as she could, hoping she would be able to sustain the effort, pulling on all her reserves. The blood was pumping, she was breathing hard, but she was doing it. A few miles later she looked over her shoulder and realised he was no longer there. Streich had been unable to keep up the pace. Yet it was not over. Wilcox's bicycle gears malfunctioned and she had to hide herself behind a bank where there was enough streetlight to do a temporary fix. With 100 miles to go, all she had to do was stay laser-focused, make no more mistakes and keep riding. Maintaining that consistent pace she had been cycling for days. She couldn't get a flat tyre. She had to make sure she didn't 'bonk' because she had zapped her energy reserves. Finding that delicate balance between pushing herself as hard as she could and having enough in the tank to make it all the way. She still felt like she was losing her mind but, before she knew it, the end in Yorktown was in sight.

There was no fanfare, no sea of cheering fans, nothing was marked, she just needed to hunt down the monument that signalled the finish line. The road for the final section was rough, everything hurt and she was still convinced that something would go wrong. She hit a building site and had to find a way around, unsure even where the route was. Then it appeared. Wilcox had made it and declared herself 'officially cooked'. A small crowd cheered as she reached the monument after cycling 4,200 miles in 18 days and 10 minutes. She had climbed 69,000 metres over some of the most impressive mountains in the US. All alone with no help, wearing the same T-shirt and shorts she started out in. This petite, inexperienced cyclist – at least from a race perspective – had become the first woman and first American to win the race. She beat the previous women's record by three days and achieved the second-fastest ever time. Someone handed her a beer, but feeling 'pretty horrible' she instead had a drink of water and collapsed in a heap, grateful to no longer be sitting on a bike. Her victory was a clear one. Streich crossed the finish line two hours later.

Part of Wilcox's success had been that she did not quit, she adapted her plans, always learning as she was cycling. It was not going well initially, the leaders were far in front keeping a faster pace but once the terrain got tougher in Missouri, she hit her stride. For the first week her knees were hurting but that passed and she felt far more comfortable once she was in the mountains. While others were unable to maintain the speed they had generated initially, Wilcox was the steady tortoise gaining ground on the hares. She has her own theories about why women may be better suited to endurance. There are very few who show up to the starting line of the ultra events she has excelled at and that also means they have less experience. 'But what I see out there is the guys lose their minds. They can't eat enough and we're smaller and tend to carry a bit more weight so we don't hit our physical limits quite as quickly. You can live off your own body for a while.' In her experience, women cyclists are good at handling pain and dealing with whatever is thrown their way. Decision-making is such a key part of it, especially when you're sleep-deprived or lacking fuel. That's when you make an error. 'Maybe it's also because the men are more driven by ego from the start.' She has seen male competitors start a two-week race like it's a two-hour event, launching into a full-out sprint. 'They go out super hard and then they just die or they blow up and then make a bunch of mistakes and end up ten places back. The woman's version is usually more like they are 10 paces back and then they catch the group.' She just wishes there were more women showing up to the race, ignoring the doubters and proving to themselves they can place high up just doing it their way.

...

Mental and tactical considerations aside (more on this in Chapters 15 and 16), Wilcox may have had a specific physiological advantage at the end of that race when she was pedalling around, whilst her nearest competitor was too tired to keep up. It is something you can see by looking at a biopsied sample of muscle tissue under a microscope. It has been shown time and again that males have larger, stronger, faster and more powerful skeletal muscles than females. Yet power is not everything, especially if it runs out. Under a microscope, the fibres that make up muscles are not uniform. They have certain characteristics depending on the job they need to do. Scientists know this because they do fun experiments in laboratories stimulating muscles with an electrical current to get them to contract and see what happens. One type of fibre is called 'fast-twitch' or type II and they are designed for short powerful bursts of energy. By contrast 'slow-twitch' or type I fibres are very resistant to fatigue. They do not tire as easily and can keep doing the same action over and over. These are the types of muscles that hold our skeleton up without us even noticing. The soleus muscle in the calf has lots of them because of its vital role in posture and standing. It is constantly active because it has to pull on the skeleton to stop us falling forward. Type I muscle fibres are also the ones that are triggered first at the start of a movement before the type II fibres are recruited for extra power. Type I fibres help with endurance; cycling, running or swimming over long distances because they do not easily fatigue and can keep going for longer. Fell runner Wendy Dodds (see Chapter 4) once subjected herself to a muscle biopsy which showed she had a very high proportion of slow-twitch fibres relative to fast-twitch. It explained why she had never been a sprinter despite her standout athletic ability over multi-day mountain adventures.

...

There are differences between females and males in the make-up of their muscles. This is often oversimplified as women having more slow-twitch muscles and men having more of the fast-twitch variety. It is more accurate to say that on average females have a greater distribution of slow-twitch fibres. This means proportionally women have a ratio where type I muscle fibres are more dominant than type II – which is the complete opposite of men. If you look at a cross-section of a bicep, men and women have similar numbers of muscle fibres overall. But in males the diameter of the fibres is bigger – and that is particularly the case for the fast-twitch type II fibres. Proportionately, a greater part of a sample of a male bicep is made up of the fast-twitch component. Ultimately, the muscle will tend to be larger because of the fatter diameter of the fast-twitch fibres and because of the size of those fibres, it will contract more quickly. It is the reason why on average males are 40 per cent more powerful in their muscles, particularly those in the upper body.

The slow-twitch, type I fibres are really important in endurance events because of how they are built. They have more of the tiny capillaries that keep them supplied with a steady oxygenated blood supply. They are also packed with mitochondria – the tiny factories within cells that carry out chemical reactions to provide energy. It is the perfect recipe if you want muscles that will work continually without burning out. Plenty of studies have found that women tire less quickly when doing specific muscle contractions over and over on repeat. Under experimental conditions, these static contractions of the arm or lower limb muscles are done in such a way that it takes power out of the equation. Sandra Hunter, who is the lead author on the consensus review on sex differences in sport (see Chapter 7), has conducted many of these studies. For example, doing a specific contraction by engaging the arm muscles at 50 per cent of an individual's maximum, having a short rest and doing it again. Women doing this were able to last three times longer than men, she reported in 2001. When repeating the contraction for six seconds, with four seconds rest for as long as they could manage, the men lasted an average 8.5 minutes while the women lasted for 23.5 minutes. The exercise where you sit against a wall as if held up by an invisible chair and see how long you can last is another example where significant sex differences are generally seen. In fact, females have been shown to be more fatigue-resistant in multiple muscle groups. But to what extent these fatigue-resistant characteristics observed in a laboratory environment provide an advantage in an ultra-endurance event out on the trail, hill, road or sea is another question.

Guillaume Millet, a professor at Jean Monnet University in Saint-Etienne, France, has spent the past two decades looking at muscle fatigue in extreme exercise and the limits of human endurance. Rigorously scientific in his approach, he is one of the few researchers who not only looks at sex differences in this area but also takes his work out of his university building and into the mountains. Over more than a decade he has done multiple studies at the Ultra-Trail du Mont-Blanc (UTMB) race series in the Alps. Whether women are better at endurance depends on how you look at it, he explains. You could just stand at the end of a long race and see whether a man or woman wins outright. Most of the time that is probably a man. But he has a different way of considering the question. If you define endurance as the ability to not slow down as the distance increases, then women are better, he says. He knows this because he has studied it very carefully. Millet is happy to debate the evidence all day long, and happy to be proven wrong. His goal is to remove as much bias as possible from his experiments. Take for example the question – does the gap in endurance performance between men and women reduce as the distance increases? That does not have a simple answer, he explains, because it depends how you look at the statistics. If you just compile data on winners of all the ultra races men will come out top. There will be outliers in some races – women who are top of their game and come first – but this way of looking at the data does not take into account who else is competing. If you only compared the top male and top female athlete in any given year in ultra running you could conclude the gap between the sexes remains the same as seen at shorter distances, he says. A different approach would be to look at the average across everyone in a race or series of races. This could well bring you to the opposite conclusion that women can close the gap over extremely long distances and maybe even surpass their male counterparts. But here you are not accounting for the fact that women are only a small proportion of the field – say 10 per cent – and those that do take part are likely to be fairly good at it and pretty dedicated just by virtue that they are there. Here the statistics are also skewed.

To get around this and create as true a picture as possible, Millet used a dataset of more than 38,000 trail running races held from 1989 to 2021 across 221 countries. This spreadsheet recorded distance, elevation, technical level as well as anonymised date of birth, sex and nationality for 1.8 million runners. From this vast repository he found 7,251 pairs of men and women that had the same relative performance over short distances – between 25 to 45km – and he looked at what happened to their speed when they ran up to 260km.

This approach showed clearly (and robustly) that the gap between the sexes decreased as the distance increased. In short, for every 10km run, men's speed dropped by 4.02 per cent but women's fell by 3.25 per cent. His graphs show decisively that as the distance grows along the bottom axis, the large gap between men and women disappears. The lines come together. It remains true whether you look at the elite (who start further apart) or nearer the back of the pack. This is the fairest evidence yet that women do indeed have greater endurance capacity, he says, that they are 'closing the gap'. He has not done the same analysis for cycling but suspects the pattern would be the same. While there are multiple factors to consider, one he has studied is that women seem to have muscles that are more resistant to fatigue.

He has done the experiment many times, both in the laboratory but also most interestingly in athletes after they have competed in the UTMB. These brave participants have already run one of the world's most demanding and fast ultras before they show up to be further investigated by Millet and his band of researchers. They test the impact of the race on muscle fatigue by asking their guinea pigs to keep contracting their muscle over and over again until they are too tired to continue. After a race like the UTMB, where athletes have run up and down many thousands of metres, there is a large decrease in what their muscles can manage. It is important to distinguish whether this is due to the muscle itself or the ability of the nervous system to keep telling the thigh or calf muscle to contract. To pick apart what is happening, his research team stimulate the nerve feeding the muscle with an electric current. Millet describes this as 'not comfortable but not torture'. By repeating this on relaxed and contracted muscle they can differentiate between central fatigue (the nervous system) and peripheral fatigue (the muscles).

The first time they did this in 10 men and 10 women who had completed a 110km UTMB run – it was shorter that year due to bad weather – they found that there was no difference in central fatigue, but the women they tested had less peripheral fatigue. 'The difference was really at the muscle level'. A few years later they decided to do the experiment again to check it was not just a one off and whether the same would be true of shorter ultra distances. So back to the UTMB they went, where athletes have a choice of different race lengths. They thought they might get a different outcome with shorter distances – say 40km – but in fact the outcome was the same. Women had measurably less muscle fatigue whichever distance they looked at.

In the more recent study, they also asked the participants about their approach to the race, trying to elicit how competitive they were feeling before they started. Millet freely admits it is an unscientific approach, but his team were interested in exploring whether there was a link between how hard an athlete may be pushing themselves and how tired their muscles were at the end. What they found suggested that the men had intended to push themselves more and the women less so, and perhaps that could also influence muscle fatigue. Teasing out the factors involved and how they interact with each other will take more research. Millet also has plans to interrogate the race data in more detail to look at pacing strategies, especially when moving on the flat or up and downhill, to see how that links to the differences in endurance and muscle fatigue. Other researchers have pointed to the ability to recover as being another area ripe for more investigation.

...

Lael Wilcox has not had her muscle biopsied. She does not know what proportion of her thighs and calves are made up of slow-twitch fibres but there is one aspect to her story that suggests she has a unique ability to withstand fatigue. Every rider taking part has their own way to get ready to cycle more than 4,000 miles across a continent. For Wilcox, she simply rode her bike to the start of the Trans Am race in Oregon from Anchorage in Alaska. It's a journey she has taken a few times. She had been doing some part-time work in a bike shop and they were supportive of her next adventure. Cycling is how she gets about, travels and sees new places. It means she can visit isolated villages along the way that not many people get to see. It is not a short trip. Over three weeks she rode down to Haines, before catching a ferry to Bellingham and cycling down the west coast of America to her destination. It is a journey of more than 1,000 miles in itself. It helped to prepare her mind and body for so much time in the saddle. She was also getting used to being outdoors and because she was on a new bike it meant she could test everything was working. By the time she began the Trans Am, everything had come together. 'At the beginning it all seems so impossible but you just have to stick with it. That determination and consistency got me there in the end.'

In the years since, Wilcox, now aged 37, has continued her adventures as well as working to get more girls riding bikes in her home state. She has run programmes to collect, mend and donate bikes to schoolchildren as well as teach cycling and bike repair skills. Her driving force is to give young girls the confidence to start riding their bikes. Wilcox finally has a sponsor which takes the pressure off. And she still prefers the mountains, 'I like climbing,' she grins. She has seen a growth in women taking part in cycling yet racing has remained largely dominated by men. 'At this point, it is still a pretty open playing field for women to turn up and just give it a go. Maybe they're not the fastest, but they have other skills and they end up surprising everyone. I like the fact that it's still such a wild sport and anyone can just show up and give it their all.' Being better at enduring through tired muscles is just one of many reasons those women could repeat Wilcox's success. It's one of a myriad of physiological factors that could explain why women may be faster the longer the distance.

11.
FAT GAINS

The stocky woman with broad shoulders and dark tousled hair sat in the freezing cold water tank. A band of laboratory staff stood over her feverishly making notes on their clipboards. She smiled a broad warm grin and looked over at the clock on the wall. Almost two hours had passed. Fighting the urge to move as the cold water rushed over her skin, Lynne Cox calmly asked the scientists if they had everything they needed. They nodded, and the young woman, dressed in nothing but a bathing suit, stepped out of the tank. The experiment had gone to plan but the results had once more astounded the research team. The 20-year-old student was undergoing tests at the Institute of Environmental Stress at the University of California, Santa Barbara, where researchers were investigating body type and physiological reactions to cold water immersion. During one test Cox swam in 10-degree Celsius seawater for four hours while a doctor followed her on a canoe, regularly taking her body temperature. Expecting her core body temperature to drop, due to the cooling effect of the cold water, the researchers couldn't believe the results. After four hours in the water Cox's core temperature rose from its normal level of 36.4 to 38.8 degrees Celsius. They hadn't seen anything like it before. The young woman was responding in the opposite manner to all test subjects whose core temperature dropped the longer they stayed in cold water. Cox had mastered the art of acclimation, with her body heating itself up to a higher-than-normal body temperature. This meant it didn't have to work as hard to stay warm, enabling her to create more heat as she swam.

Fascinated by her ability to acclimatise, the research team continued their experiments on Cox from 1975 to 1979. The cold water swimmer was a unique specimen but her response to chilling temperatures also told a wider story about women and fat utilisation during long durations of exertion. During this period Cox attracted the attention of a world hypothermia expert, Dr William Keatinge, of the London Hospital Medical College, and was flown to the UK for further tests. Keatinge had been studying an Icelandic fisherman who had fallen overboard and survived by swimming to the shore, a painful five-hour journey through icy waters. The national hero had sat in Keatinge's tank for 60 minutes as his core body temperature gradually declined. The next step was to compare his results to a female swimmer. And so, at the age of 22, Cox found herself sitting in a tank of five-degree Celsius water at the University of London. But this time the lab team had to keep lowering the water temperature as Cox's body heated it up. They did everything they could to prevent the water from warming, including creating a current to stop a layer of warm water forming close to her body, and asking her to sit still. Despite their best efforts the temperature rose by one degree. Cox was an anomaly, but she was also proof of the power of nature, nurture and acclimation and the vital role played by body fat.

Born with fine downy hair covering her body, Cox's mother joked that her baby daughter looked like a seal. Premature and weighing just five pounds, Cox quickly put on weight, growing larger and stronger than the other kids. Worried that she was bigger than her peers, her parents got her tested and discovered she had an efficient metabolism which lent itself to endurance sport. With her parents' encouragement Cox soon realised she loved being in the water more than on land. It was in her blood after all. Her grandfather Arthur Daviau was a long-distance swimmer who swam across cold-water lakes in Maine, something her mother also did during childhood. As a medical corpsman in the Navy attached to the Marines, Cox's father spent much of his early life on the sea. While her doctor grandfather strongly believed genes had a great bearing on people's health and development, what Cox inherited more than anything was her family's passion for swimming. Her younger brother was an open water swimmer who swam the English and Catalina Channels and while Cox was breaking ultra-swimming world records her sisters were playing water polo for the US team. The family were so dedicated to swimming that they moved 3,000 miles across the USA from the mountainous New Hampshire region on the east coast to coastal California on the west, when Cox was 12. This enabled the children to receive the best training possible under the guidance of an Olympic swim coach, Don Gambril.

While she was not the fastest in the pool, what Cox did better than any of her siblings was to excel in cold water, training her body to not only survive, but thrive. The expectation of her parents was to simply do the best she could, but for Cox this meant being The Best. Not the best female swimmer, but the best swimmer. Using her physical advantage as a larger woman with higher body fat content than her male competitors, she spent years acclimatising to frigid temperatures. When out of the water she would wear light clothes and walk around in bare feet and flip flops all year round. As she headed to the beach for a training session she strode out in her swimsuit, never taking a towelling coat to keep her warm. Cox would not have been seen dead in a DryRobe and was rarely spotted in a swimming pool. Rather than wearing a wetsuit, neoprene socks and swimming gloves, she simply waded into the cool sea water in her swimming costume, her only accessories being a pair of goggles and a cap. She even forwent the use of grease commonly slathered on sea swimmers, claiming it would neither keep her warm nor make her safe. The smell of the ocean grease, made from wool fat, would attract unwanted attention from sea creatures, and make it difficult for her emergency team to pull her from the water, she argued. Her own body was more than enough.

...

It began, in 1971 at the age of 14. Stepping onto the fine orange sands of Seal Beach, California, Cox stood in front of the familiar crashing waves, her short-cropped hair gently buffeting in the breeze. Staring at the popular pier-walkway in the distance, she prepared for her first epic swim. She was part of a squad of four teenage swimmers vying to become the youngest team to ever swim the 21-mile Catalina Channel which separates Santa Catalina Island from the southern California mainland. The fresh-faced foursome strode confidently into the swell and set off. Stopping only to sip warm apple juice and nibble on oatmeal raisin cookies, they executed the crossing in 12 hours and 34 minutes. Along with acclimation, finding the right fuelling method was all part of the endurance puzzle for Cox. Throughout her years in college she constantly gathered fuelling ideas from other long-distance athletes learning that ultra runners favoured avocado on bread or peanut butter and jam sandwiches. While these supplies worked well in the heat, they did not prove effective in cold, wet, salty water. Instead, Cox experimented with liquids settling on warm peach and pear juice which had the dual benefit of giving her a sugary energy boost whilst soothing her tongue and throat, swollen from the salt abrasion.

Seeking a solo challenge in 1972, aged just 15, Cox shattered the men's and women's English Channel world records from England to France with a time of nine hours and 57 minutes. Despite her success, the achievement was undermined by reactions of disbelief. 'People were absolutely astonished and I had telegrams coming from all over the world sort of surprised. And people said I was lucky because I had really good conditions and that's why I was able to complete the swim,' recalls Cox, more than five decades later. On the contrary, the swim had been anything but easy since the only means of navigation was radar rather than following the straight line of a GPS tracker. Cox had no idea how far off course the radar and currents would take her, or how long she would be swimming. She simply took the approach 'you just keep going until you get there'. Shortly after she crossed the Channel her record was broken by a male swimmer, Davis Hart. This turned out to be a blessing in disguise. 'It meant I had another goal to go back and break his time. And it turned out that I swam three miles further, and the conditions weren't as good as the first time, and I still swam 21 minutes faster and regained the overall record. I proved to myself that yes, a woman or a girl can be faster than any man.'

This was just the beginning of Cox's phenomenal ocean career. Cox was the first person ever – female or male – to swim the Skagerrak Strait between Norway and Sweden in 1976. The 19-year-old's six-hour 16-minute achievement received nothing but a small write-up in the local paper with the headline 'Lynne Cox Sets Record'. The same year she set another first. Swimming in 5.5 degree Celsius water, in nothing but a swimsuit and cap, she traversed the Strait of Magellan, in Chile, battling against a nine-knot cross-current. Swimming in icy waters became her forte. She became the first person to swim between three of the Aleutian Islands in Alaska. Next she tested her limits swimming the three lakes of New Zealand's southern alps, setting records for swimming at high altitude in extremely cold temperatures. She became a pioneer in sea swimming spending as much time planning the logistics as she did training.

Keen to show what the human body was capable of she made a career of swimming crossings no one had ever attempted before. In 1977, she braved the shark and sea-snake-infested waters of the Cape of Good Hope to become the first person to swim 10 miles around the southern tip of Africa. All of this was just a warmup for her main event in 1987 – attemting to become the first athlete to swim the 2.7

miles Bering Strait between the USA and the Soviet Union, during the height of the Cold War. Eleven years in the making, Cox had sought permission directly from the Soviet leader, Mikhail Gorbachev, for the gesture to bridge the distance between the two countries.

At the age of 30, with the support of Alaskan senators behind her, she emptied her bank account and travelled to Little Diomede Island in the middle of the strait. It was a risky strategy because she didn't receive permission to do the swim until the day before it was planned to go ahead. Even more of a gamble was what would happen to her body when she swam in a swimsuit through the glacial ocean that sat at the gateway to the Arctic. On 7 August, she set off into the fog to find out. 'The water was six degrees Celsius and within the first mile it dropped to three. I could physically see the changes. My fingers were turning grey, my face was bleaching out, my crew was very concerned I'd go into hypothermia. Keatinge and Dr Jan Nyboer from the University of Alaska were there in a support boat monitoring my temperature. I'd also swallowed a thermal pill created for astronauts to measure my core temperature whilst swimming. To check if I was OK they would roll me onto my back and I'd do backstroke for a bit. But I was getting too cold, so I told them to stop. I just needed to swim otherwise I would cool down too much, lose heat and never get it back. It was really challenging, and we were really in the unknown.

One concern was if I went into severe hypothermia, I wouldn't be able to grab onto the float or the boat because you can't control your fingers and you don't feel your arms. But I never thought I should stop, I just relied on the experts to tell me if I needed to get out, because I wouldn't have been able to tell and with severe hypothermia, I could die.' As Cox crossed the border a Soviet skiff approached asking if she could swim a further 300 metres to a welcoming committee on Big Diomede Island. Longing to get out of the freezing water but desperate to make a connection with the Soviets, Cox reluctantly agreed. When she reached the snowbank at the shore the icy rocks made it impossible for her to climb out. Cox thrust her hand out of the water and three Soviet soldiers grabbed her arm and lifted her out. For the first time in 48 years the border was open.

Underestimated throughout her twenties for simply being a woman, Cox understood that her sex actually gave her a three-fold advantage. Firstly, her fat ratio meant she was able to maintain core body temperature in freezing waters. This layer of additional warmth kept Cox alive when she swam in -3 degree Celsius water off the coast of Disko Bay, Greenland, in 2007. 'Swimming the Bering Strait was like going to the moon, but the swim off Greenland was like going to Mars. A few degrees in temperature made an incredible difference. There were icebergs in the water, the only reason it didn't freeze was because of the salt and currents. But I wanted to see how far we can go as human beings and what's within our capabilities. We are so fragile yet so strong.' Those same fat stores were sufficient and efficient enough to sustain her over marathon swims more than six hours in length. 'The extra body fat means if you can't stop to eat, because you are going to be seasick, or you're breathing in fumes or tasting salt water in your mouth, you have stores to give you energy. It's not optimal but it's enough to keep you going.' Thirdly, the fat gave her more buoyancy making it easier to glide through the sea even as she fatigued. In Cox's case she had a special kind of buoyancy, described by sports physiologist Dr Barbara Drinkwater as 'neutral buoyancy.' This meant her body density was exactly the same as seawater, with the proportion of fat to muscle perfectly balanced so she neither floated nor sank. Cox was at one with the water.

To date Cox is the only athlete to have ever swum the Bering Strait, and she holds more than 50 world records and firsts to her name. Her lifelong achievements and resilience to the cold are unquestionably extraordinary but she also reflects a lesser-known phenomenon. In the world of cold open water swimming, women are usually faster than men over long distances. Competitive ultra swimming, often referred to as marathon swimming, is any event longer than 10km. There are rules setting it apart from ordinary open water swimming which mean athletes cannot stop, are not permitted to wear a wetsuit and cannot have any assistance during the race. Several studies have been conducted on the Triple Crown of Open Water Swimming, the UTMB of the seas. These are the three most well-known marathon swims which incorporate the 21-mile English Channel Swim, the 20.1-mile Catalina Channel Swim in the United States and the 28.5-mile Manhattan Island Marathon Swim. The fastest completion time for the triple was set in 2005 by Marcia Cleveland, then 32 years old, and it still stands today. The American swimmer, who is a member of the International Marathon Swimming Hall of Fame, was slower on the English and Catalina legs than an Australian, Benjamin Freeman, who holds the second-fastest triple crown record. It was the longer stretch through the East, Harlem and Hudson River around Manhattan Island where Cleveland excelled, finishing the loop an hour faster than 19-year-old Freeman, who was 13 years her junior.

It is only relatively recently that scientists have begun studying sex differences in marathon swimmer performance. In 2011, a team from the University of Zurich analysed the English Channel's best times from 1900 to 2010. Women achieved similar or better performance times than men. The World Open Water Swimming Association also examined results from the English Channel and found the average female completion time was 33 minutes faster than the average male time. Women took the lead more significantly in the slightly longer Manhattan Island Marathon swim, performing 12 to 14 per cent faster than the best men, according to 30 years of results scrutinised in 2014. A similar study on the Catalina Channel times from 1927 to 2014 concluded the fastest women were faster than the fastest men. And not by a small margin. The fastest woman ever was 22 minutes quicker than the fastest man. The biggest differences were found when comparing the annual fastest women and men, with the women pulling ahead by an average of 53 minutes. Data in amateur swimming also shows a marginal sex difference between women and men in open water. Data from 117,000 participants taking part in Great North Swim events in northern England from 2008 to 2023 reveal the average time of males is faster than women in shorter open water distances. But once events stretch beyond two miles the average female time eclipses men during some swims. At the 2022 Great North Swim 10k, the field was made up of 61 per cent men and 39 per cent women. Despite there being fewer females, their average time was marginally quicker. Similar results were recorded at two miles and 5km distances.

Clearly something is giving female swimmers an advantage. These women, like Cox before them, are not the lithe, sinewy athletes that line up at the start of an ultramarathon. They are stockier, curvier and heavier. They have more body fat. Triple crown researchers (studying those who have swum the English Channel, Catalina Channel and the Manhattan Island Marathon) have surmised women marathon swimmers had between 30.7 and 31.3 per cent body fat while in comparison the men had between 18.8 and 20.2 per cent. While the women's body composition was almost one-third fat, it accounted for just one-fifth in the men. This higher fat mass made the women more ergogenic in the water, meaning they were more efficient. Since fat has a lower density than muscle and is distributed mostly in the buttocks and thighs of women, compared to the abdomen of men, it increases buoyancy and reduces drag.

Fat also provides lifesaving insulation against the cold when swimming without a wetsuit in waters where temperatures can vary from 15 to 21 degrees Celsius. This is especially important in longer distances such as the Manhattan Island Marathon Swim where athletes are in the cold water for extended periods of time. Swimmers with higher body fat are able to stay longer, and perform stronger, in cold water compared to those with lower body fat. If you take temperature out of the equation, men in pool swimming events are still faster than the best women. However, the longer the pool swim the smaller the gap. This is partly due to the third fat advantage afforded women. Thanks to higher levels of the hormone adiponectin, women are more efficient at metabolising fat because they oxidise it, turning it into energy, at a higher rate than men relative to their body mass. This is believed to be oestrogen-mediated and can be used to enhance male performance.

When Canadian researchers gave 12 healthy young men oestrogen supplements their lipid oxidation increased both at rest and during endurance exercise. With significantly higher oestrogen and adiponectin levels women can make better use of fat energy stores than men over extreme distances. This is because ultra endurance relies heavily on oxidative metabolism for the efficient use of glucose and lipids to fuel muscle movement. Women, particularly young females, are especially good at using mitochondria (the powerhouse of cells) to take little molecules of fat and break them down. In essence, the fat gives muscle cells energy. The ability to better mobilise and oxidise lipids during ultra distances is highly beneficial and can often lead to a late metabolic second wind. Over 24 hours, regardless of the exercise undertaken, women exhibit 24 to 56 per cent greater fat oxidation compared to males. While this is a biological function designed to support pregnancy and feed young infants, it may have become an evolutionary advantage to facilitate endurance (see Chapter 9). Women carry between five and 10 per cent more body fat than males, which becomes a big advantage the longer you exercise. Nick Tiller, an exercise scientist at Harbor UCLA, who studies physiological responses to ultra marathons says fat is the most important ultra-endurance fuel, because you can burn through carbohydrate stores in a couple of hours. 'Someone doing an ultra marathon would run at a much slower pace than they would a marathon or other race of a shorter distance. This means they can burn more energy-dense fats. If you're working at a much higher intensity, you have to rely more on carbohydrate. If women are better at burning fat than men at a given relative intensity, which they are, this could potentially be one advantage for them in ultra-endurance events.'

Conversely, if an athlete is less efficient at burning fat (as is the case with men), then they will burn relatively more carbohydrate. This becomes a hindrance in longer events because the body has a limited internal store of carbohydrate, Tiller explains. Fat is also more energy dense than carbohydrate, containing more than twice as many calories per gram, so being able to access this store is more efficient and staves off early-onset fatigue. Carbohydrates, when consumed in high amounts over a long period, can cause gastrointestinal distress such as abdominal cramps, diarrhoea, nausea and vomiting. So, females' lower dependence on carbs could be advantageous. Being more substrate efficient and having a smaller body size, and stomach, also means women need fewer calories in general which again mitigates debilitating stomach issues common in ultra endurance. Taken together, these differences give women a metabolic advantage during exercise of extreme duration, whether on land or in water.

For swimmers like Cox, fat provides the triple crown of warmth, buoyancy and energy metabolism. Even in her sixties enjoying her life as an author and motivational speaker, Cox is still able to swim for hours in the Californian sea each day, enjoying the 'balmy' 16-degree waters. On dry land, it is the power of fat metabolism that can give women the edge in running, cycling and multi-sport events. They don't just have more fat; they are also better at using it (see slow-twitch muscles Chapter 10). For women fat is nature's energy source with a vital role to play in motherhood; the ultimate endurance feat of them all.

12.
TOUGH MOTHERS

Chelsea Sodaro is preparing for the biggest race of her career so far. She is on the island of Kona in Hawaii to compete in the annual Ironman World Championships. The pinnacle of the triathlon calendar. Through school and college, Sodaro had been a middle-distance runner, competing in national cross-country and track competitions. Watching the 2016 Olympics on television, injured and feeling dejected because she had been unable to qualify, her husband had suggested she switch to triathlon. She initially laughed at the idea, but gave it a try and was hooked. The wins came almost immediately. Triathlon competitions offer a range of distances and she quickly moved up to half Ironman which covers 70.3 miles (113km) over a swim, cycle and run. Less than five years after her first event, Sodaro has doubled the distance again. She is about to compete in her second full Ironman against the best female athletes in the world. It seems strange that this elite event has not been renamed Ironwoman for the women's race, which is run separately to the men. Her mind is racing but as she looks out over the stunningly Hawaiian lush scenery of Kona towards the bright blue sea she spots a rare double rainbow. It must be a good omen. In the past month, her training has finally come together and all she can do is give her all.

On race day, against all odds and expectations, Sodaro crosses the finish line first, almost eight minutes ahead of the second-place triathlete. In eight hours 33 minutes and 46 seconds she swam 2.4 miles (3.9km), cycled 112 miles (180.2km) and ran a full marathon (26.2 miles or 42.2km). It is a stunning achievement for the rookie athlete. It is not just the distance that makes this Ironman race one of the most challenging and gruelling one-day sporting events there is. Kona's waters are choppy with exhaustingly large swells. After conquering the seas, those taking part then have to charge up the beach to the rhythmic sounds of Hawaiian drumming, speedily transitioning to the road bike. Cycling past excited crowds, black lava flows and towering volcanoes, competitors must endure hours in intense sun. It is a hilly, island course and the wind can be problematic. The cycling alone would beat most people, especially in the Hawaiian heat. Yet when the triathletes have carefully placed their bike on the rack, they have to change shoes and run. At pace. For Californian-born Sodaro, this was a very quick run. Slightly slower than some of the others in the water and on the bike, she needed to make up time. By mile eight she was in front, her lead increasing with every mile. The others could not keep up. By mile 19 she was a full five minutes ahead. Her final time as she flew over the finish line with her hands in the air is the best the Kona race had ever seen, bar one.

Sodaro's win captured the media's attention far outside the niche world of endurance triathlon. She did not have a professional contract, was little known in the sport, and was first US woman to win the race in a quarter of a century. She was the underdog. Yet by far the main reason she hit the headlines was that just 18 months previously she had given birth to her first child. How had she managed this after the physical demands of pregnancy and childbirth? It seemed that she had come back a better athlete than before. How was that possible? The 33-year-old had chosen to have a baby during the Covid-19 lockdown when races were not happening. It seemed like the ideal time. During her pregnancy she had kept training under the careful guidance of an experienced coach despite suffering badly from morning sickness. At times she would have to stop a session on the stationary bike in her garage to vomit. She kept working and stayed as focused as she could. While she may have been an unlikely winner, she did not come unprepared to the World Championships. Her coach, Dan Plews, a former triathlete based in New Zealand, had competed in this very race. She knew how the course and conditions would feel and she had a plan to execute. In an interview just moments after she won, Sodaro said: 'My mind is a little bit blown right now, but I think this is the culmination of things being right in my life and having perspective. The greatest gift at the finish line is my little 18-month-old.' Looking back on the day from her home in Colorado where she recently moved with her family and now three-year-old, Sodaro has had time to reflect more fully. 'It was one of those days where the stars aligned. Things were going my way and I was making the right decisions.'

It was by no means a perfect race. A lot can happen in eight hours. A third of the way into the cycle section, she lost all the nutrition she had brought to fuel the ride. But where once she would have panicked, she literally took the setback in her stride. 'I am an emotional racer and person and the one thing I think motherhood has changed for me is my ability to handle chaos,' she says. 'It was very validating. Like my life's work coming together.'

...

The win that day in Kona added Sodaro's name to an increasing list of female athletes who come back seemingly stronger after pregnancy. Paula Radcliffe began running again just 12 days after giving birth to her first child, winning the 2007 New York City Marathon nine months later. On the track, US sprinter Allyson Felix won her 12th gold at the 2019 World Championships 10 months after having her daughter by emergency caesarean section. At the same games, Shelly-Ann Fraser-Pryce made history by becoming the first mother

(her son was then two years old) and the oldest woman to win the 100-metre sprint. UK heptathlete Jessica Ennis achieved gold at the 2015 Beijing World Championships 13 months after her son was born and nine months after she was able to resume training. She pointed out there were 10 mothers in the GB team for the most recent 2024 Paris Olympics. So many that for the first time at an Olympic Games the athletes village had a creche. Yet when she competed in Rio in 2016, she had been the only one. In tennis, Serena Williams won the French Open 16 months after having her daughter. She was wearing a black bodysuit that she said at the time made her feel like a 'warrior princess' but was medically necessary to prevent blood clots because of post-birth complications. She admitted after the event that she had been pregnant when she won the Australian Open in 2017.

The numbers may be increasing but it is not just a recent phenomenon. In 1991, the Scottish runner Liz McColgan showed her drive and sheer determination in the World Championship 10,000-metre final where she systematically burned off every other athlete on the track to take the gold medal nine months after giving birth. At the time, advice on training in pregnancy was completely non-existent, but through listening to her body, the 23-year-old was able to run right up to the day she went into labour. Her daughter, Eilish is also now a 5km and 10km runner, holding the British and European records. A study looking at the effect of pregnancy on 42 elite to world-class runners, published in the journal Medicine and Science in Sport and Exercise in 2023, found that most were exercising again by six weeks and had returned to their usual amount of training by three months. Almost 60 per cent of them ended up with better personal best times, the Canadian researchers found.

In the world of ultra sport, this book has already mentioned several women who broke barriers or records after having children. Eleanor Robinson (Chapter 4) had three young children when she first started out in ultra distance. Jasmin Paris (Chapter 1) broke the Spine record when her daughter was just 14 months old and still breastfeeding at night. Sophie Power (whose story is explained in Chapter 18) showed the elite ultra-running world just how sexist it was by breastfeeding her three-month-old at an aid station on the Ultra-Trail du Mont-Blanc after being refused a race deferral. She has since gone on to represent Great Britain at the 24-hour running championships and more recently broke the record for running the length of Ireland, her three young children providing the reason for even attempting it. The US ultra-running legend Pam Reed was overall winner of the Badwater 135-mile race in Death Valley, California, in 2002 and 2003, having had three children (and two stepchildren): she was in her early forties at the time. Every single one of the athletes mentioned here attracted intense media coverage that made much of the fact they were mothers, 'bouncing back' quickly from pregnancy and birth. In some cases, they were still breastfeeding. The expectation is this can't be done; they have achieved the impossible. Yet what if the female ability to adapt to the demands of pregnancy is not a disadvantage, but a secret weapon.

...

There is some evidence that ultra athletes may have easier pregnancies. Exercising in pregnancy is known to reduce the risk of high blood pressure and gestational diabetes. But being an endurance athlete may also confer other advantages in coping with pain, particularly during labour. Those used to ultra endurance have already developed techniques to handle pain. Researchers have also theorised that oxytocin, or the love hormone, which is released both in labour and during intense exercise may help people remember pain in a more favourable way. Many women are routinely managing pain throughout their teen and adult lives due to menstruation. It is often assumed that for this reason women handle pain better than men. Laboratory studies do not support this. Yet experienced ultra women will often have coping strategies that can help them manage the labour process. Carla Meijen, a Dutch sports psychologist, has written about how anyone can use those strategies to support an empowered birth. It is about understanding what you can control and what you cannot. To be flexible when something is not happening how you expected it to. Meijen says: 'The experience of pain in childbirth is of a different level but at the same time, knowing you have managed and encountered difficult situations and you have tackled them successfully can be a bit of a confidence boost. There is also the idea about learning from that pain going back into sport.' Meijen has also seen athletes who were used to controlling all aspects of their lives suddenly have to adapt to uncertainty when they have a baby and their timetable is no longer their own. 'For ultra athletes they just have to accept "if I don't go out for training now, I'll miss my chance to do it" and the conditions might be less than perfect but I can do this. If you think about self-efficacy as the ability to be successful in a task, you are building up a lot of flexibility in the self-belief that you can do something.'

The North Face-sponsored ultra runner Stephanie Howe knows all too well that it can take time to come back to a new normal after pregnancy. In her labour, after four hours of pushing, and the threat of a caesarean section, the midwife said to her: 'What are you doing? You are an athlete, don't fight the pain, use it.' It was exactly what she needed to hear and her son was born soon after. Originally from the US but now living in Chamonix in France, Howe sees in her peers a parallel with efficiently managing kids and work and home with the demands of ultra racing. She is a single mum and has to plan her childcare very carefully. 'It does translate well to an ultra where you're juggling all these things and you just cope. It doesn't throw you off'. With a two-and-a-half-year-old, she is still learning how to meld motherhood, her work as a scientist and ultra racing. 'Pregnancy did change my body and I still don't feel fully recovered but it isn't about bouncing back it is about moving forward with what you have and accepting it is going to be different.' She was surprised by how long that took physically, she admits, but the hardest shift was psychological because she had to come to terms with leaving this infant for hours at a time to train. 'I don't think you understand unless you go through it, how much it changes you.' Pre-pregnancy, Howe won her first 100-mile race, the infamous Western States, leading the pack from 30 miles in. 'I still get tingles thinking about that.' But her second proudest moment was her first big race back after having her son. 'I just bombed, I don't even know where I finished, maybe in the 40s or something but I didn't even care, I came to the finish line and saw him through the crowd and that was a really amazing moment. He is here and I'm still competing.'

After pregnancy, some of this ability to return to the sport and continue winning medals and breaking records may be down to having an inspiring new motivation, a renewed sense of mental toughness, or something to prove. Yet it also poses a question as to whether pregnancy itself confers some advantage, particularly for an endurance athlete. After all, isn't pregnancy the ultimate endurance test? The female body goes through dramatic changes in the 40 weeks from conception to birth, a process that encapsulates the fundamental adaptability and resilience of the female body. The moment a fertilised egg implants in the wall of the uterus, a series of signals trigger the drastic changes needed to support a pregnancy. The menstrual cycle stops and over the next few weeks the embryo begins to develop rapidly, forming the structures that will ultimately become organs, including the brain and heart. The placenta, a whole new life-sustaining organ, begins to grow in these early weeks. By the end of the first trimester at week 12, the foetus is about the size of a plum. Outwardly there may be little sign that the woman is pregnant but already she may have had weeks of morning sickness (which does not just happen in the morning), sore breasts due to changes to prepare for breastfeeding, many more trips to the toilet to urinate, heartburn and quite intense levels of fatigue.

In the middle part of pregnancy, known as the second trimester, many women report that their energy starts to come back. Sickness and nausea can lessen. Women with a healthy pregnancy often say that this period is the best they feel physically during the nine (more like ten) months. It is not without its issues, including swollen hands and feet, ligament pains in the expanding belly and hips, backache and dizziness. But in general, pregnant women usually feel less tired and that extreme tenderness in the breasts can ease. While they start to look pregnant, it is still fairly simple to move about, at least compared to the final few weeks. This is also a time of intense change to the growing foetus. The organs mature and move to the right position, genitals develop, hair begins to grow and the baby moves around a lot, which the woman will start to feel. In size, the baby grows from peach to cauliflower. Then in the final stretch, in weeks 28 to 40 (aubergine to pumpkin) the baby gains weight, and especially fat, and fully develops the lungs that will allow it to breathe, as well as undergoing rapid brain development. The placenta is the organ that enables all this to happen. Most people think of the placenta as the connection between the mother and foetal circulation, but it does much more. It essentially functions as the lungs, digestive system, kidneys, and liver for the growing baby but also produces the hormones that help the female body adapt to pregnancy, keep the immune system from attacking it, initiate labour, and prepare for breastfeeding. The placenta also controls the maternal metabolism and the level of glucose needed in the mother's blood to provide a constant source of nourishment for the foetus and itself.

One of clearest associations between pregnancy and ultra-endurance sport is the increased metabolic demand on the body. One study which set out to map the ultimate limit of human endurance by analysing elite running and cycling events found that the metabolic rate achieved during the longest endurance challenges is comparable to pregnancy. Herman Pontzer, professor of evolutionary anthropology from Duke University in North Carolina, and colleagues, analysed data from the Tour de France cycle event, an arctic trekking competition, and the Race Across America involving six marathons a week for months. They discovered the longer the event, the harder it was to sustain a higher metabolic rate. The body can only do that for so long. For a marathon you can push this energy-burning capacity to more than 15 times what it would normally because you only need to do that for a matter of hours. For the Tour de France which lasts around three weeks, it is 4.9 times higher. Ultimately – and this was shown in the Race Across America – any metabolic increase settles at around 2.5 times higher than the resting metabolic rate. The limit is probably due to what the human digestive system can cope with rather than capacity of the circulation or muscles. What was striking to the researchers was the similarity to pregnancy where the metabolic rate or energy use peaks at 2.2 times higher. 'Prior to our paper, most people were talking about maximum sustained energy expenditures as a sort of one number thing, for example maybe it's four times your base metabolic rate,' Pontzer explains. 'We wanted to know how event duration plays into that.' Looking at these incredibly high energy expenditure events, they found a curve that settles around two and a half times. 'I was racking my brain as I was putting the dataset together and thinking what is the longest high-energy event we have data on, and then I realised that pregnancy fit the criteria. When we looked it fell exactly on that line.'

As well as dramatically increasing metabolism, every organ in a woman's body changes when she is pregnant. Everything has to adjust to cope with large fluctuations that at any other time would indicate serious health problems. The biggest adaptation is to the cardiovascular and respiratory systems, so that the body can cope with the vast increase in metabolic demand. By week 34, a pregnant woman has an extra 1.5 litres of plasma, the fluid part of the blood that carries nutrients, hormones, proteins, water and salts around the body. Red blood cells have also increased by 18 to 25 per cent. To keep all this circulating, the heart has to work harder. So it gets bigger and stronger. In the first trimester, cardiac output – a measure of how much blood has been pumped in one heartbeat – grows by 20 per cent and in the second trimester peaks at 50 per cent. Most elite athletes can only dream of these kinds of endurance adaptations. Achieving this magic combination of greater cardiac output, lower blood pressure at rest and increased red blood cells is the whole point of endurance training, especially at high-altitude. In a well-conditioned pregnant athlete, research has also shown an increase in VO2 max (the maximum oxygen uptake) by the end of their pregnancy. This improvement in how the body makes use of oxygen may also shorten the process of giving birth. Researchers have estimated that with every five per cent increase in VO2 max, there is a 28-to-33-minute reduction in active labour time. The heart rate rises during pregnancy to an extra 10 to 20 beats every minute but blood pressure does not, in fact it goes down slightly. During pregnancy this boost in cardiorespiratory fitness is all driven naturally by hormones rather than intense training sessions.

...

The question for female athletes is whether this endurance advantage can be harnessed to boost physical fitness and conditioning through training while pregnant – and how long it lasts afterwards. It may be that these changes are what helped Sophie Power run through her pregnancy and complete the UTMB three months later while breastfeeding. Never mind the metabolic changes needed to sustain pregnancy, lactation requires even more in terms of extra daily calories. Yet this cardiorespiratory benefit is likely to be pretty short-term. The increased blood volume is thought to return to normal within a couple of months. For those athletes tackling challenges once their baby is a year or more old, the specific advantage conferred by higher metabolism may well have disappeared. Yet researchers think the higher levels of oestrogen produced during pregnancy along with some other adaptations could provide longer-term benefit. This is just a theory and difficult to study from an ethical perspective. Cara Ocobock, a human biologist and anthropologist at the University of Notre Dame, Indiana, whose research into evolution and endurance (see Chapter 9) started her thinking about the physical benefits of pregnancy, says we just don't have the answer. 'No one has actually studied this, but if we think about going to Mount Everest and eventually not getting as lightheaded as you used to be, your body does acclimatise. In pregnancy it is acclimatising to the additional calorie burn, extra blood flow, ectetera, and then once the stimulus is removed you would see a decline. If someone like Sophie Power picks up and goes back to her running that stimulus is still there and so it should maintain. Theoretically, this makes sense, but we don't have the data to back that up.' The role of oestrogen overall – pregnancy or not – in providing females with an endurance advantage should not be underestimated, she adds. 'Oestrogen is the underlying force behind all these changes.'

...

It is important to be clear that not all pregnancies are straightforward and for some women returning to race fitness can be a very steep uphill battle. Not least because of the potential for injury as a result of relaxed ligaments and changes to the pelvis. The textbooks can explain what is supposed to happen, but pregnancy varies between individuals and among pregnancies for the same woman. After her third baby, Power had a check-up with a specialist physiotherapist who identified she had a pelvic organ prolapse. After three babies and a lot of running it is perhaps not too surprising – and it is a common condition. Power had to build up very slowly, undertaking a strength programme which included pelvic floor exercises. She also had to hold back on the running, which she admitted was very frustrating. But sticking with the plan was motivated by the desire to 'still be running when I'm 70'. Knowing when to hold back is extremely important postpartum. There are 'return to running' guidelines to help women in this period, who may have separation of abdominal muscles or incontinence. Some may easily keep to the training they were doing before, but equally others may have the opposite experience. 'You accommodate to how you feel,' says Ocobock. 'It is the same thing that people would tell you about periods when you have to compete. You just find ways to accommodate.' Of course, labour itself places huge demands on the body and can take days. A caesarean section, if needed or chosen, is serious abdominal surgery that takes weeks to recover from. Then there is the exhaustion of caring for a newborn. Notwithstanding the profound psychological challenges related to the mental strain of new motherhood, a changing sense of self, and postpartum depression.

Practically, returning to training can seem almost impossible in those early days when the baby does nothing but feed. Yet if anything, this makes the achievement of those mothers who surpassed expectations all the more impressive. Sodaro's new coach, Dan Plews, was immediately up for the test of seeing how she could train through her pregnancy. A father of young children he was fully aware of what pregnancy and having a baby entailed. As a professional athlete, Sodaro had a support system in place. She had a set-up at home which meant she could train. And she was carefully monitored by Plews who tracked all her data. She also had insight into her own ability that meant when it felt harder in the later stages, she eased off. Training is usually the part where she could trust the process. Yet in pregnancy, while recovering and caring for a newborn there had been a lot of twists and turns. For an athlete used to controlling every aspect of her life, it had been a difficult and daunting time. Just how difficult only became apparent after her win. During her pregnancy and after her daughter's birth, she had been suffering from crippling anxiety and intrusive thoughts that later turned out to be a manifestation of obsessive compulsive disorder (OCD). It had been made worse when her baby struggled to feed and gain weight. She had to make trips to the paediatrician and lactation consultant every other day. Her daughter was later diagnosed with a tongue tie and a milk protein allergy. 'I felt like I was a capable person and this was something I should be able to get done,' Sodaro said. 'I've never worked harder at anything in my life than trying to breastfeed.' Sodaro was probably back to pre-pregnancy levels of fitness by five months postpartum, but training itself was not easy. She had ongoing problems with urinary incontinence when running. Eight weeks before Kona, she had been ready to throw in the towel, exhausted juggling work and childcare while her husband was working shifts as a firefighter. She was pushing herself harder than she ever had before.

...

There remain some unknowns around training in elite athletes during pregnancy. Research has shown that even high-intensity training can be safe and beneficial but the upper boundaries of this, especially for those elite athletes who push themselves to their very limits, needs further investigation. What is certain is that pregnancy is not some fragile state where women have to be wrapped in cotton wool. There is strong evidence that moderate exercise in pregnancy is beneficial and guidelines around the world now recommend this. Pregnant women are encouraged to exercise even if they did not before. It is a hard cultural shift to make after many decades of advice to the contrary, explains Linda May, an exercise physiologist at the University of East Carolina who studies active pregnancies. Back in the 1980s, only women used to exercise were recommended to do any, and then only for a maximum of 15 minutes a day. The most recent recommendations from the American College of Obstetricians and Gynaecologists are similar to those for the general population advocating 150 minutes per week of moderate-intensity exercise. Such activity has been shown to lower resting heart rate, increase cardiac output, improve fat metabolism, cut the risk of gestational diabetes and can alleviate aches and pains that come with growing a small human. The body is already doing this adaptation, but exercise boosts its impact. May's research has shown that exercise also benefits the baby. 'People have looked at resistance or strength training, just aerobic training, some type of concurrent training and shown it's all fine, it is safe, and mum and baby both benefit. The guidelines have progressed to say basically you should be doing the same as the average person.' May points out that pregnant women get the same benefits from starting to be more active as anyone would. 'If they were naive to exercise, they're just adapting to pregnancy and exercise simultaneously and our amazing bodies are able to do that.' Studies have also shown that women who manage to be highly active during pregnancy in general have an easier (and shorter) time in labour with fewer complications. They may also have a faster post-delivery recovery.

However for the endurance athlete this recommended level is far below their usual physical activity level and is therefore not particularly helpful. Ryanne Carmichael, an exercise physiologist at Plymouth State University in New Hampshire in the US, became interested in this topic when she was pregnant herself. As a former amateur triathlete who had moved into cycling, she was used to a lot of training. For women like her there was a big gap in the recommendations. 'I was an avid endurance competitor, but no one knew what I should be doing. I asked my doctor if I could do a plank, and he said: "What's a plank?".' In 2021, she wrote detailed guidelines for coaches based on the current evidence while noting that training for endurance sport in pregnancy presents some unique challenges. 'I am happy with that as a resource but there also needs to be something for postpartum because while the changes you see in pregnancy are great for fitness, then you have a newborn and that is the difficult part. Your physiology might be such that it improves your performance but not on three hours sleep.'

Carmichael describes the changes to the cardiovascular system during pregnancy as 'magnificent' and points out they can persist. 'We do see that anecdotally in professional sport for instance, like with British cyclist Lizzie Deignan, who won not that long after having her baby,' she says. 'If you come into pregnancy already trained like these endurance athletes have, with really high plasma volume, really high cardiac output, then they get pregnant and get this huge boost in cardiovascular ability. It persists but it persists during a time that for a lot of women they may not be able to take advantage.' It is highly individual and it is important not to get sucked into a message that all women should be doing an Ironman after giving birth, she says. 'It is an important distinction, especially with things like parenting and pregnancy because what is easy for you isn't necessarily easy for someone else, not because you're stronger, just because of the circumstances.'

Sodaro, the victor at Kona, describes the first year of motherhood as 'brutal'. She is unsure if she would take the same intense approach again. More than anything she wants new mums to just be 'kind to themselves'. But she also stresses the importance of taking time to pursue things that 'light us up' because it makes us a better parent. After pregnancy, Sodaro, like many women, was at her most vulnerable. She was physically and mentally broken. She had severely disrupted sleep, undiagnosed OCD, and was recovering from the endurance of pregnancy and birth. Yet she was still expected to carry on. Sleep be damned. Like all mothers, she had to find the reserves, even when at her most exhausted.

13.
WHO NEEDS SLEEP?

Jamie Aarons pulls out a dehydrated chocolate brownie pack to use as a pillow on the bare hillside. It is more comfortable than the bicycle tyre she recently used. Once her nap is over, the brownie inside has turned deliciously warm and gooey. Perfect for a wake-up snack. It is surprising how people find comfort in the middle of an adventure that has stripped away all luxury. Aarons is running – and hiking – up a remote Munro (a peak over 914 metres or the nice round traditional number of 3,000 feet) in Scotland. She is exhausted. She is four weeks into a challenge to climb 282 Scottish mountains in one continuous self-propelled push. Aarons was up before dawn after grabbing a few hours of sleep in a small tent left by the team supporting her. Quickly downing a high energy shake of the kind elderly people are given in nursing homes, she has been moving ever since. Now, many hours later, the tiredness is catching up with her and there is still a lot of ground to cover before she is done for the day. Almost falling asleep on her feet, she decides to stop for one of her infamous 'micro naps'. This is her superpower. If tired enough she can fall asleep almost immediately, like turning off a switch, and wake up again five or ten minutes later, recharged and ready to go. Since she began this adventure, which involves running, walking, cycling and kayaking for a total of 2,576km, she has slept in all manner of strange places.

This ability to handle sleep deprivation is the driving force behind 43-year-old Aarons' attempt to break the overall Scottish Munro record. Others who have done the self-propelled challenge may have relied on speed, but she knows she can make up ground in other ways. This is all about using her specific strength to her advantage. It proved to be a winning strategy. In June 2023, she completed the feat in 31 days, 10 hours and 27 minutes, knocking 12 hours off the previous record held by an ex-marine. However you carve up the statistics, they are impressive. Aarons covered 1,315km on foot, 830km by road bike, 370km by mountain bike, 49km on her gravel bike and 11.6km by kayak. The 135,366 metres of ascent may not mean much in isolation, so her team worked out this was equivalent to climbing Mount Everest almost 16 times. In one particularly efficient day, she ticked off 14 Munros. All while being endlessly bitten by Scottish midges, those highly irritating mini mosquitoes that swarm in huge clouds in summertime.

For the quiet social worker who lives near Loch Lomond, the attention after the Munro record was overwhelming. The media loved the fact that this middle-aged woman had beaten the record held by a tough military man. She quickly put a stop to this narrative, saying it undermined both their achievements. In reality, the previous record holder, Donnie Campbell, was one of the first people she told of her plans and he turned up on one of the last Munros with his wife and dog to cheer her on. Journalists from the BBC website to niche running blogs also focused on the fact that Aarons averaged around four hours sleep in every 24 hours and not necessarily in one block. And they were right to. When the idea of the Munro round first pinged into her mind, Aarons knew sleep would be her secret weapon. A key tool in her arsenal as a female endurance athlete. Everything was set around her ability to keep going without much rest.

Aarons first had the idea of taking on the challenge while listening to a podcast interview with Campbell. Campbell was in a different class to Aarons physically: he was an athlete; incredibly fit, strong and fast. But when he was asked how he approached his daily recovery, he mentioned that he had at least eight hours sleep a night. It lit a spark; a niggling idea that would not go away. Aarons recalls: 'I realised I couldn't remember the last time I got eight hours of sleep. It got me thinking that there's more to something than just innate speed, here is the potential that I could tap into my own strengths.' It took two years to plan the challenge and for Aarons, the motivation was never really to beat Campbell, but a chance to test herself and to raise money for charity along the way. The idea was cemented when a dear friend and fellow runner, John Kynaston, died from a heart attack at the age of 61. He had been the first person she had told of her possible plans, even before her partner. He didn't laugh or tell her not to. He had been an inspiration to her when she first started trail running, an embodiment of the camaraderie that hooked her into the sport. One of the reasons she now spent all her spare time joyfully roaming the hills around her home. So when he died, the fact he had been supportive somehow turned this vague idea into a reality. The world was also beginning to emerge from Covid-19 and a homegrown adventure gained extra appeal.

Originally from California, Aarons had been a competitive swimmer in her youth. Running was not really her thing. She'd done the New York marathon once but had not caught the bug. It was only when she moved to Scotland two decades ago that she discovered trail running and loved the accompanying self-sufficiency, navigation and friendship. Many multi-day events and adventure races had taught her above anything else that she was good at handling sleep deprivation. 'It's not that sleep isn't important to me; I'm not Margaret Thatcher standing up and saying that I thrive on four hours of sleep a night,' she says. But doing ultra races alongside other competitors who were struggling had made her realise she had a 'weird ability' to cope, when others could not. 'I did an adventure race with a team of lads who were a decade younger than me who were really struggling when it came to the sleep. I was dying trying to keep up with them on the move, but when it came to sleeping, I had that sort of ability to micro nap and recover, scaffolded by my childlike sensitivity to caffeine.' For the Munro challenge, it meant she could look at a route that was not reliant on crossing a road or an access point in order to sleep in a campervan or hotel. Knowing she was perfectly capable of getting enough rest in a tent or even a basic bivvy – best described as camping without a tent – she could be far more flexible in completing the challenge. She added in extra kayaking sections because she enjoyed it more than cycling round a loch. (Most of all the challenge had to be fun.)

Friends took time off work to come and run or cycle with her, to carry kit, set up camp and essentially keep her going. The final plan, after two years of recceing, doing Munros individually, and recording everything in an enormous spreadsheet, accounted for six hours sleep a night. A week in, this all went out of the window.

Aarons estimates she probably did get six hours rest a day if you count stopping and sitting but the actual sleep quickly dropped to four after an unexpected Scottish heatwave slowed her down. For a couple of days they switched to running in the cooler nighttime weather, but that hadn't worked. She had got stuck in a low inverted cloud that made navigating much harder and everything was taking longer than expected. She needed to claw back time. 'I thought if I'm an hour longer on the hill I'll just have to sleep an hour less'. From a hormonal point of view, she suspected and was proved correct that the long hours of summer daylight in northerly Scotland would make it easier to wake up more naturally and keep going. The worst moments were when she would sleep in the dark in a van that had been kindly donated and kitted out with a new mattress. 'It was super cosy and amazing for sleeping in but the van didn't have windows and it was pitch black inside. One of my friends still says she's never felt like such a horrible human being than trying to get me out of that bed. I sleep with a stuffed cow and taking it off me to get me up was one of the worst things she has ever had to do.'

Aarons quickly realised if she didn't feel like she would fall asleep in an instant, stopping was a waste of time so she kept going. She is acutely aware she could only pass out on the side of a hill because there were people there to look out for her and wake her up. There were other times when she had an extra hour or two because her body was telling her she needed it. 'The scariest point as you would expect, because it's quite similar to when it happens when you're driving, was when I was on the bike. One time I distinctly remember being suddenly just overcome with sleepiness and just so struggling to keep my eyes open. I was with a friend and we were going downhill so we were actually going quite fast and I made us stop and lose our momentum because I realised I was officially a liability to both myself and potentially my mate,' she adds. 'Life's too short to make it shorter because I'm being an idiot who is too stubborn to stop.'

...

Aarons is not the only female endurance athlete to use sleep to their advantage. Jasmin Paris also did so to great effect in her Winter Spine record (Chapter 1), despite hallucinating wildly. Lael Wilcox also cut her sleep when she realised she was gaining on the front rider in the Trans Am race she ended up winning (Chapter 10). Anecdotally, women say they are more used to disrupted sleep – with or without children in the mix – and therefore can handle it better, retaining their ability to make decisions and do that all-important self-care and fuelling. In studies, women will rate their sleep quality as worse. They also report more monthly fluctuations in their sleep with more frequent waking, bad dreams or nightmares, or insomnia in the week leading up to and the first few days of their period. Studies on female athletes have also shown they subjectively feel like they have worse sleep overall. Sleep of course varies greatly between individuals and also changes over the life course, and is affected by both physical and mental health. When scientists look at this objectively by connecting subjects to a machine that measures different stages of sleep, women do not seem to have as poor sleep as they think they do. In general, studies suggest that women need more sleep than men, with the Sleep Foundation figures indicating that women get 11 minutes more sleep on average. Women also tend to spend more time in deep sleep and are quicker to fall into REM sleep – the phase where dreams happen. There are many possible social and biological reasons why women feel they have worse sleep. The phrase 'increased caregiving responsibilities' is the researcher's way of noting that women are often the ones who get up in the night to deal with waking children as well as dealing with the associated 'mental load'. Women are 40 per cent more likely to suffer from insomnia, research has suggested. Females are also more likely to suffer from restless legs syndrome, with twitchy limbs keeping them awake, most likely due to oestrogen.

Yet the scientific literature on sex-based differences in the ability to handle sleep deprivation paints a mixed and muddled picture. It is possible to find separate studies claiming that both men and women handle lack of sleep better. Circadian rhythms – those natural sleep-wake patterns over a 24-hour period – have an important role in regulating female reproductive hormones as well as testosterone in men. On a chronic level, regularly working night shifts has been shown to disrupt metabolism, cause gastrointestinal problems and impact mental health as well as being linked with cancer and cardiovascular disease. Given that many have children, women may well be more affected by the disruption of their normal circadian rhythm over longer periods of time. Yet extrapolating what has been shown in the laboratory into the real world is difficult and researchers are still trying to unpick what this all means. A deep dive into this topic published in Sleep Medicine Reviews in summer 2024 pointed out that part of the reason that so much remains unknown about sex differences in sleep or ability to cope with disrupted sleep is that all too familiar refrain that female participants are under-represented in the research.

When it comes to the concept of using sleep deprivation as a strategy in endurance events and whether women have an advantage, the research 'is very inconclusive', explains Jessica Mong, professor of pharmacology at University of Maryland School of Medicine. What scientists are starting to understand, she says, is that while sleep is important for overall health in the long term, the sort of extreme sleep deprivation that happens in an ultra race does not have much impact on your cardiovascular, metabolic or energy needs. Finding the physical reserves to continue in those circumstances does not have much to do with sleep. But there are numerous studies which do show cognitive disruption in the short term, including impaired decision making. 'I do wish we had more data on the sex differences in that,' Mong says.

Earlier in her career, Mong discovered that oestrogen influences the switching on and off of genes that relate to sleep. Ever since she has been doing work in the laboratory to try and work out what is happening. Much of this is done in rats and she explains that when their oestrogen level is at its highest their circadian rhythm shifts. They get up early and if they have a running wheel in their cage, they just start expending all this energy for 24 hours and then it's all back to normal. In the wild, they would be out looking for a mate. 'They have this sense of endurance' and do not feel the need to sleep. For Mong it raises the question of whether this is an evolutionary adaptation that has somewhat persisted in women. In short, it suggests females may be more resilient to sleep deprivation. 'When we started our experiments on what oestrogen is actually doing to the sleep circuitry, we found that if we sleep deprived a rodent, I mean, really sleep deprived them for 12 hours, when their oestrogen levels are high, it doesn't affect them. They're like, whatever, give me something that's really going to bother me. Their control counterparts without oestrogen become aggressive, angry, and when we allow them to go back to sleep, they sleep for 18 hours.' The animals with oestrogen get back on their circadian rhythm quickly, with only a short recovery sleep.

One aspect researchers are considering is whether ovarian hormones in women who have given birth and have not experienced postpartum depression but are very sleep-deprived are somehow helping to reduce that sleep debt. 'With oestrogen I like to think about it like credit card debt,' Mong explains. 'As we stay up throughout our day our sleep debt rises and we're buying more time. At some point our debt becomes so high that we really do need to pay it back and the way we pay it back is by going to sleep.' It is essentially impossible for an individual to stay awake for days. What researchers have found, with rodents at least, is that when oestrogen is in play, the sleep debt or that need for sleep is lower and there is a lot more room for those animals to be up and active. 'We don't have any evidence for humans, but my guess is that it is probably going to be similar and what we're trying to do is figure out how it is allowing the brain to function at a higher level.'

Genetics could also play a part in whether someone is particularly good at surviving on less sleep. People – female or male – can be predisposed to being short sleepers or long sleepers which is why sleep experts are hesitant to say that everyone needs eight hours sleep a night. 'We need to think about this in terms of sleep homeostasis, how much consolidated sleep an individual needs to feel rested. For some it can be as little as six or seven hours, four is a little extreme, but it could be that genetics has a little bit to do with someone's ability to do that,' says Mong. When it comes to Aarons and her power naps, she may also have an ability to reach that deep restorative sleep more quickly than most, which is helping her feel better even with very short stretches of shut-eye. If you are able to power nap and get to deep sleep quickly that will clear out those neurochemicals in the brain that are building up, giving you a boost.

Aarons is an intriguing example to those who study the science of sleep. Carissa Gardiner has just completed a PhD in the Sports Performance, Recovery, Injury and New Technologies Research Centre at the Australian Catholic University. Within a team that does a lot of research around sleep and athletic performance, her work focuses on the impact of substances such as caffeine and alcohol. In general, she notes, it is really only chronic lack of sleep that will impact physical performance. The acute periods of no sleep that an endurance athlete will put themselves through will probably not make much difference to their strength even if subjectively it feels harder. Gardiner also points to the cognitive impact. One study found that sleep restriction in healthy adults to four or six hours a night for two weeks significantly diminished their ability to carry out cognitive tasks. This tracks with endurance athletes who say that their ability to make a decision disappears, so they forget to fuel properly or change kit and deal with blisters or niggles in the same way that they would if they were firing on all cylinders. Something like navigation could absolutely fail.

The part of Aarons' story that made Gardiner sit up the most is the description of herself as having a 'childlike sensitivity to caffeine', which meant she could wake herself up really effectively. 'That is really interesting because there is a genetic component to this. You can be a slow metaboliser, essentially sensitive or insensitive to caffeine and it would be good to know where she would fall in that category.' On the question of whether an endurance athlete could try to train themselves to handle sleep deprivation better, Gardiner explains that you can 'normalise' functioning with less. 'So if you're used to getting five hours of sleep per night, then you can make that feel normal,' she says, but that normal will be at a lower level of cognitive performance than you were: 'That is your new level of function'.

Cheri Mah, an expert in the relationship between sleep and performance in elite athletes at the University of California San Francisco, has advised ultra athletes on their sleep strategy. She agrees it is possible to some extent to get used to a lack of sleep. Studies have shown that reaction times decline, but then level off. At the other end, Mah also points out that even after a night or two of recovery sleep, you're not fully back to 'normal'. 'We don't necessarily think that you can train yourself to do better with sleep deprivation, but you can get by.' Yet ultra athletes who need to be awake for long periods may well be a self-selecting bunch. They only do it because they know they can handle it, Mah suggests. When she is preparing athletes for a period of time when they will not be sleeping, including one cyclist recently racing from Canada to Mexico, she advises extending their sleep in the weeks before. So, if you normally do well on eight hours a night, try getting nine instead. 'I don't really like the term like 'sleep banking' because of the perception that you can surplus sleep and draw from it, which I don't believe is supported, but you can pay back your sleep debt to be at a very minimal level. Studies do suggest that that will minimise the detrimental effects that will happen when you know you're going to be short on sleep.' Mah is also a huge fan of power naps and has recommended this as part of a planned strategy going into a lengthy ultra challenge. 'There is research to show even as short as 10 minutes can be beneficial for improving alertness. Really, the sweet spot is more like 20 to 30 minutes.'

Whatever enabled Aarons to plough through her Munro record with such little rest, some of it is probably explained less by the amount of sleep she 'needs' and more by her ability to cope with the situation, Gardiner believes: 'This ties in with mental fatigue, but potentially she's very mentally resilient.' Aarons admits it never once crossed her mind to quit. In the final week of the month-long challenge, she had crippling foot pain that turned out to be from an infected internal blister. It slowed her dramatically, but it was just one more thing to deal with and that made her look forward to the periods she had on the bike. 'I had confidence in my own resilience and my own knowledge that the lows, however low, get better. You don't know when or how or why, but that low is going to pass, and I just need to persevere through it.' She has mind games she plays with herself when things get tough, doing some mental arithmetic to keep her brain ticking over and focused on something else. But it was also her experience of doing multi-day events and being out in the hills for long periods at a time that gave her some of that in-built mental resilience that may in part help her to overcome deep fatigue and be present in the moment.

Aarons said: 'One of my absolute highlights, which somewhat ironically came on the back of one of the worst experiences of the entire month, was coming down off the last Munro on Knoydart, which is very remote. I was with a friend who was struggling a bit on the descent. The terrain was horrific. I can't overstate how bad it was, it was really quite dangerous with deep holes and it was very slippery and craggy. We parted ways once it got dark because we could both be seen with head torches and I ran on to the loch. The midges were unreal, it was just grim. A friend had left a kayak and paddle and buoyancy aid on the shore. I got into my boat and was initially terrified that I was going to have this 4km crossing of just being eaten alive. But as soon as I got onto the water, the midges disappeared, and everything was so still, just like glass. The moon was bright, and I switched off my head torch and I just paddled silently on my own across the water. It was one of the most peaceful and surreal and amazing moments. I could see the silhouette of the hill I was going to do next in front of me. On the opposite shore, my partner Andy and some friends had borrowed a pizza oven and got it going so from about a kilometre away I could smell the food. It was an out-of-body experience and felt so much more amazing coming straight after such a low point. After refuelling we walked up a hill and as the sun rose, the memory of that low point was now long forgotten.'

The science as it stands cannot tell us if women have an innate ability to handle sleep deprivation. For Aarons, sleep was the clear strategy that enabled her to knock half a day off the record, despite hobbling towards the end. Surviving on a couple of hours sleep a night plus power naps, she was able to make decisions, function and beat the record, she did the challenge again – and she has no plans to – she would adapt further. This would mean using a different bike and being more flexible in the complicated logistics her team had set up. 'I know I had it in me to do it in under a month and there are people out there who are much faster than me on the move, or who are equally capable of being strategic on sleep or even using a different pacing strategy. They could use another strength that I don't have, so breaking my record is definitely possible if everything works in your favour.' As Aarons reflects, there are plenty of other tools women can employ in their attempts to break ultra-endurance records.

14.
THE PACING GAME

A lack of confidence is not something Sabrina Verjee struggles with. Despite being left on the bench when all the sporty kids had been picked by their mates, she never let it knock her self-esteem. A British outsider with dark skin and short-cropped hair, who was neither black nor white, Verjee threw herself into every challenge. With a French mother and a father of Indian heritage born in Kenya, Verjee always felt different, but it never held her back. Short in stature, but large in fearlessness, she was not the stereotypical woman battling the odds. Her lack of athletic ability during her early school years rapidly evaporated when she attended Charterhouse, a quintessential English boarding school, to complete her A levels. Days were filled with rock climbing, football and cross country, where she learnt that she was not the fastest, but she could definitely run the furthest. This innate ability was drawn from a special kind of tactical restraint which would serve her well in future sporting challenges. In the meantime, she secured a place at the University of Oxford, where she soon joined the rowing squad. Self-assured, Verjee naturally saw herself as the 'most reliable and attentive member of the team' with a good power-to-weight ratio but soon discovered she couldn't tolerate the internal politics. Leaving the squad, she found a more welcoming home in the modern pentathlon team, developing her skills in fencing, swimming, show jumping, pistol shooting and running. She may not have been an outstanding competitor, but Verjee still proudly celebrated her half-blue status. This was awarded to athletes achieving a good standard but falling short of the higher grade of a full blue. Unsurprisingly, before she had even graduated, Verjee, who described herself as a 'bright student' courted by various banks, was offered a highly competitive role with Credit Suisse First Boston in London's Canary Wharf financial district. But it wasn't enough. Verjee longed for a role where she could use her brain while simultaneously embracing the outdoors. Not content with working in an office, she soon quit her lucrative banking job to pursue a career as a rural veterinarian.

···

Her hearty confidence continued throughout her twenties as she sought greater thrills and entered the world of adventure racing. She competed in British, Irish, Spanish and French mixed-sex teams, which were typically one woman and three men, to meet the 'mixed' criteria. She was typically unphased by the testosterone-infused environment: 'I don't think a lot of women would be as ballsy as me to go and race with guys you don't know.' These multi-day races involved navigating unmarked wilderness courses via foot, mountain bike and kayak. Here, she honed her skills as the reliable tortoise, pacing consistently rather than tearing off and then crashing. Verjee unequivocally believed she had 'far more experience than the men', was just as capable at map reading and was an expert in sleep deprivation. But the men did not see it like this, and she was continually thwarted by her male teammates. 'God forbid anyone put a map in my hands, that would never be allowed. Which is just utterly ridiculous. Just because of your gender you don't get to do any of these things. You're supposed to just shut up and do what you are told. I definitely felt that in adventure racing. And I raced with a lot of teams.'

Ultimately, Verjee decided she would be happier on her own doing ultra running, where her 'natural aptitude for endurance and self-reliance' could be harnessed. She launched herself into the fell running scene, moving from the flatlands of Bedfordshire to mountainous Cumbria, home of the lakes and fells. As she began to make a name for herself in the UK ultra running world, her exuberant confidence did not go unnoticed. In June 2019, she led the Montane Summer Spine Race from start to finish, becoming the first ever female athlete to win the 268-mile race outright. This was just six months after Jasmin Paris won the winter version of the same event (see Chapter 1) in arguably harsher conditions. Despite this groundbreaking achievement, she failed to win an elusive spot in the top 10 of Ultra-Trail du Mont-Blanc (UTMB) Chamonix, the world's most competitive 100-mile race. She came 21st. Verjee claims she was never running for a top 10 position and was just 'out for fun'. Damian Hall, British ultra-running royalty who has numerous Fastest Known Time records, a Winter Spine Race win and a fifth UTMB podium place to his name, can't hold back his admiration for Verjee's self-esteem. 'Sabrina just has striking confidence, more so I think than Beth Pascall and Jasmin Paris, the latter who I coach. Even though those two have a top 10 at UTMB, and Sabrina I don't think troubles top 10, she's got incredible confidence.' This unflinching confidence, that she could compete with the best, improve her times and work on her weaknesses, eventually led Verjee to take on 'the ultimate prize' – running the Wainwrights.

...

Bog snorkelling, cheese rolling, caber tossing, welly-wanging. Britain has a knack for creating quirky sporting contests. Tackling the Wainwrights is another arbitrary pursuit which grew out of a series of 1950s picture books. Written by Alfred Wainwright between 1955 and 1966, the seven pictorial guides feature 214 peaks in and around the Lake District National Park in Cumbria, north-western England. Known locally as fells, these peaks were chosen by Wainwright as mountains to conquer. There is no criteria for mountains to be a Wainwright, other than they were written about by him. The peaks come in a number of shapes, heights and sizes from the tallest Scafell Pike at 978m to the smallest Castle Crag at 209m. Since the arrival of Wainwright's Pictorial Guide to the Lakeland Fells 'bagging' all of the peaks has become a popular hobby for hikers and trail runners. Most people attempt to tick off the peaks over a lifetime, with the more ambitious tackling them over a year. But few have tried, and succeeded, in running the round in one go. The first recorded continuous Wainwright was achieved in 1985 by Alan Heaton in nine days and 16 hours. To be a Fell Runners Association ratified round, the route must start and finish at Moot Hall in Keswick but after that competitors can create their own route as long as they summit every peak. As a popular walking hotspot the trails are relatively hard-packed but depending on the route some sections involve scrambling up steep, rocky terrain. Owing to the elevation and the lack of woodland, the views are often spectacular, stretching miles into the horizon, overlooking glistening lakes and billowing grassland. Living on the doorstep of the Wainwrights in the Lake District, Cumbria, England, Verjee had her eye on the challenge for a number of years. She cut her ultra-running teeth on the mountainous Dragon's Back Race in Wales and Summer Spine on the Pennine Way, England, where she beat her nearest competitor by more than eight hours in 2019. But the Wainwrights were always in her sights and, buoyed by her Spine win, she started recceing the peaks in earnest.

She wanted to complete the Wainwrights in under six days. At the time the record was held by Paul Tierney, who did them in six days, six hours and five minutes, covering 318 miles and climbing the equivalent of Mount Everest four times. But Verjee insists she was not bothered about breaking the record, because the challenge was a personal goal. Finishing the Wainwrights Round in six days and five hours (and breaking the record) would not be enough. She wanted to finish in under six days. In fact, she was so indifferent to record breaking that she happily set off during lockdown in 2020, despite being told by the Fell Running Association that the round could not be ratified. Verjee was not driven by ego, media attention or record books. She did not want to be the fastest person to complete the round, or the woman that beat the man. She wanted to see if it was possible for her, personally, to finish in less than 144 hours. She set her own rules for the continuous round and pledged not to leave the route as others had done, to navigate entirely by herself and to respect access law and the Countryside Code, meaning she could not cut across private land and had to stick to public rights of way (unlike previous record breakers). With meticulous planning and preparation, she considered this mission possible.

While Verjee concedes men have more speed and power than women, she believes women 'can be smarter'. As someone who had always run her own race, been efficient at checkpoints and never changed her plan when overtaken by another racer, she knew that consistent pacing was her secret weapon. It was one more tool in her strategic arsenal and Verjee had to stick to the plan. A plan that was six years in the making. 'Maintaining pace was crucial, but I knew I didn't even have to think about my pace. I only really have one speed and I can do that for a very long time.' Although her pace would inevitably slip as the days progressed, she knew it wouldn't drop off as steeply as others because she was starting from a slower speed to begin with. This also had additional gastrointestinal benefits. Because she wasn't pushing her body as hard as other athletes, she was able to eat and drink regularly and avoid cramps, vomiting and diarrhoea – stomach issues that typically affect ultra runners. This pace also gave her 'staying power' and aided her mental ability to keep going and going. This efficient way of moving, and reserving energy meant she could cut back on sleep.

Finely balancing speed and self-preservation, she found her sweet spot was running four kilometres an hour. The ability to sustain even pacing, from the very first hour of her six-day adventure, came naturally to Verjee, who had always run at a consistent speed. It just so happened that she could keep going at this speed for day, after day, after day. Such evenness is not surprising when you delve into the performances of women at long distances. The running shoe testers Run Repeat have been gathering race metrics for the past decade and hold one of the largest databases of running statistics. Time and again, its data reveals that women run at a more consistent pace. The most recent stats, analysing 2.3 million marathon results achieved during 2009 and 2019, show that women are 18.33 per cent better at keeping an even pace than men. This means they burn out less often in the second half of a race. The results, taken from six worldwide marathons (Boston, Berlin, Chicago, London, New York, Paris), also discovered runners who started slower were more likely to run a more even pace than those who started faster. The classic tortoise and hare analogy in real life.

Age also impacts performance with runners aged 19 and under, 56 per cent more likely to burn out in the second half of a marathon compared to 35 to 44-year-olds. Jovana Subic, head of running research at Run Repeat and herself an ultra runner, believes ego-driven males who go out too fast striving for a short-term adrenaline fix, could learn from women how to achieve a personal best by reining it in and maintaining a consistent speed. 'What we do notice at races is that men start faster. That decision could be ego-driven, an overestimation of one's skills, but it could be as simple as being taken away by the crowd.' Put this together with evidence from peer-reviewed field studies which demonstrate male long-distance runners are consistently more optimistic than female runners, and a picture starts to emerge. Overestimation in one's ability can result in men finishing slower than their own prediction. A working paper by The University of Gothenburg in Sweden found that in a marathon men tended to overestimate their finishing time by four minutes more than women. By comparison women had a more realistic idea of how fast they could run. Although the data from Run Repeat is not publicly available, and lacks peer scrutiny, multiple peer-reviewed studies based on smaller sample sizes have established that women pace themselves better than men. Why is this? Psychology, according to Francois-Xavier Li, a sports scientist at the University of Birmingham in the UK, who believes the source of pacing consistency is likely to be psychological rather than physiological. He says: 'It is a well-known fact that women pace better than men. You could say that men receive more adrenaline and start faster. Some papers show men are overconfident and are overestimating their ability.'

Men's tendency to adopt a riskier strategy by starting too fast is well documented in the research. With more even pacing, an athlete is less likely to slow considerably in the latter stages and lose more time than they gained in the beginning. In ultra races, the stakes are even higher. By running too fast in an ultra event over six hours long, competitors considerably raise the risk of early onset muscle fatigue, energy loss and what is known as 'bonking' or 'hitting the wall'. This can make all the difference between a personal best time and a did not finish (DNF). When extrapolated to running continuously for several days, only taking short naps sporadically, avoiding complete energy failure is the number one goal. Verjee therefore, had to keep moving at a sustainable speed if she was ever going to hit sub-six on the Wainwrights.

Verjee set off to master the Lake District Wainwrights in June 2020 – with a pacing plan. Her goal was to keep moving and minimise rest. The spreadsheet was complete, the OS maps were marked and the first pacer was weighed down with extra weight so he ran at exactly the right speed. It was a stiflingly hot summer's day but this meant ground conditions were good and Verjee skipped merrily down the dry rocky slopes without fear of sliding. Lapping up the sunshine she made steady progress over the fells, picking up fresh pacers en route.

Unfortunately, by nightfall the weather had turned and before long she was scrambling up the hard steep nose of Yewbarrow, slipping and sliding through a torrential downpour. The final slog to the summit through sodden bracken was rewarded with a howling wind which then propelled her off the peak via a strong tailwind. She quickly made it back down to more sheltered ground and began changing in the waiting campervan for the next leg of the journey. Despite the challenging conditions, she was on track and feeling good. That was, until, she received a message from the assistant chief constable of Cumbria. What she was doing was illegal, he warned, she was legally obliged to return to her home once every 24 hours. Having pored over the Covid-19 rules, she didn't agree, but she also didn't want to risk being prosecuted. She halted her attempt after 24 hours. She wasn't even tired because her pacing had all gone to plan. She had run consistently and eaten consistently. But rather than being thwarted by setting off too fast, encountering impassable weather conditions or sustaining an injury, she had been stopped because a policeman told her she had to sleep in her own bed at night. Even though she wasn't planning to sleep. For now she needed to sit and wait for the next legal window of opportunity.

Fortunately, the wait was brief and one month later she was given the green light by the police. This time the attempt ended in a bittersweet victory. Three days into the route, Verjee was on target, but whilst descending The Nab she felt a pull in her right adductor on the inside of her thigh. Trying to ignore the pain she strode onwards, hiding her winces from the crew. Gradually the painful burning sensation spread to her knee and before long she had made a costly pacing error. This, combined with a lack of adequate fuelling, proved to be catastrophic in the second stage of the challenge. While steady pacing is effective in multi-day feats of endurance, this only works if the body has a continuous source of energy. Running at speed over short distances is stressful for the body and causes it to defer to the sympathetic nervous system, which promotes the fight or flight reflex in response. This is no use for running long distance because it relies on energy stored in the body which will ultimately deplete. You cannot store an infinite amount of energy. However, when running at a less intense pace under less stressful conditions, it's possible to tap into the parasympathetic nervous system which stimulates the rest and digest response. As Verjee knew only too well, the key to setting a sub-six-day record would rely on running at a slow enough pace to digest her food and benefit from the energy boost, while moving quickly enough to meet her target. This meant eating at least 300 calories every hour for the entirety of the challenge and sticking to her pace. Despite being armed with this knowledge, on day three Verjee ran too fast and ate too little, while her leg swelled up. As she hobbled down Seat Sandal near the village of Grasmere at the break of day four she gripped the arm of her pacer, grimacing in pain. It would not be the first time in this Wainwright attempt that she would use her supporters as a human crutch. Staggering through to the end, she finished in six days and 18 hours, falling short of her personal target.

Confident as ever that if she just stuck to her plan, and avoided injury, she would complete the Wainwrights in less than six days, Verjee made another dogged attempt in April 2021. This time she was defeated by respiratory failure due to the freezing, wet conditions and had to pull out after three days. A lifelong asthma sufferer, Verjee developed a wheezing so severe that she felt she was being strangled. Unable to stop coughing, Verjee hit the emergency button on her tracker and abandoned the attempt: her third. A course of catabolic steroids (to treat her asthma) and a tooth abscess later, she found herself ready to take on her fourth Wainwright attempt on 11 June 2021. Her sex bore no relevance when it came to her persistence and determination. While naysayers thought her stubbornness was misguided, Verjee was ready to keep fighting on her own terms. Setting off at a steady pace, she managed to keep the asthma at bay. Over the next five days she grabbed just a little over five hours sleep and kept on track. But with just 23 peaks and 50 kilometres to go, her right quad began to hurt substantially, causing her to slow down. This time she avoided energy depletion by eating copious amounts of cake. Verjee was comfortably within reach of breaking the Wainwrights record but was only just on the cusp of her dream of breaking six days. She had to stay awake, ignore the growing bulge in her thigh, and keep moving.

With laser precision focus, she fought off the sleep demons screaming in her head and put one foot in front of the other. Every stop had to be productive because she was now pushing the limit of her ability. With three peaks to go she was bang on schedule, and although her team were anxious, Verjee knew she was going to do it. With just a couple of hours to go a doughnut was placed in her hand, giving her legs an instant sugar boost. Savouring every last moment, Verjee bagged Brown How, the final summit. Taking a minute to soak in the achievement she even had time to pose for a beaming photograph. Then, unceremoniously, she descended the hill, content in the knowledge that she had achieved her personal goal and completed the 36,000 metre round in less than six days. There was no fanfare, media scrum or celebratory champagne. Instead, Verjee hugged her husband Ben and went home for a warm bath. On her fourth attempt, her pacing plan had finally paid off, combined with meticulous preparation and a huge dollop of confidence, sheer will and determination. She finished the Wainwrights in a new record of five days, 23 hours, 49 minutes and 12 seconds. A ready, steady record-breaking run. This momentous accomplishment demonstrated the significant role played by pacing, and how it could help give women an edge. But it is just one mechanism in a complex puzzle. Winning an ultra-endurance event is not about speed and strength alone: muscle fatigue, metabolism, sleep deprivation and biological endurance are all interconnected factors affecting the outcome. But what of psychology? Might this be the biggest leveller of all?

15.
MENTAL MYTHS

When the internet is asked to picture a maths professor, it does not conjure up a tattooed woman with long flaming pink hair. Instead, an online search shows hundreds of photos of middle-aged men, mostly wearing spectacles, or women in suits with frighteningly white teeth beaming in front of a chalkboard. No one has brightly coloured peroxide hair or a tattoo arm-sleeve of inspirational women, like Michelle Jeitler. Her staff profile at Marietta College, Ohio, USA depicts a smartly dressed brunette with pearl earrings; but that's not the real Jeitler. The ultra-running maths professor rocks up to class in a hoodie and jeans, unashamed of her dark roots growing out from underneath her neon pink locks. She explains that studying ultra-running data is not a normal activity for an Ohio mathematician and some days she must defend herself for even speaking in the company of men. Drawing inspiration from Joan of Arc, Dolly Parton, Cleopatra, Henrietta Lacks, and Ruth Bader Ginsberg – all tattooed on her arms – Jeitler is using her discipline to dig into sex differences in endurance racing. She loves solving puzzles and encourages her research students to dig into the heart of endurance myths.

Working with a maths graduate, Lexi Jobe, she investigated the claim made in the documentary Finding Traction that nearly all women cross the finish line at the Leadville Trail 100-mile race, while less than half the men complete the race. Similar declarations have been made about the UK's Dragon's Back race, a 236-mile six-day race covering 16,400 metres of elevation. Jasmin Paris strongly recalls the impact of a speech given by a veteran fell runner, Helene Whitaker, at the start of the 2015 race. 'I can't remember the exact figures, but Helene said to the room that you've got a 50 per cent chance of finishing if you are a man but if you're a woman you've got a 90 per cent chance. And it played out like that pretty much. The point she was trying to make is if you're a woman, there might be fewer of you, but you've come there better prepared. Women only sign up if they've got the self-belief and the preparation to do it. Whereas the men are more gung-ho and think they can get away with it.' Figures from the race year-on-year seem to back this up. In 2023, half of the male field did not finish Dragon's Back, while only a fifth of the women racing dropped out (15 per cent of the whole field were women). This would give credence to the view that women are less risk-averse, tend to be more prepared and once they sign up for a tough race, they are going to finish it. Except Jeitler's research showed something very different. Jeitler and Jobe pored over 66 years of data randomly sampling 30 US ultra-marathon races of at least 100 miles in length. The dataset covered a diverse variety of elevation, location, temperature and altitude. And what did they find? That there was no difference between the did not finish (DNF) rate of women and men. Even at Leadville. DNF rates were the same. The commonly held view that women are less likely to drop out of a race before the finish was not substantiated. When it came to mental capability the battle of the sexes did not have a clear frontline.

This is just one example of the myths that perpetuate the sport – and society at large. Tell an anecdote enough times and it morphs into fact. The clearest example of this is the job application story, trotted out by numerous sources during the writing of this book. According to one piece of research, men will apply for a job when they meet just 60 per cent of the essential criteria while women will only apply if they meet 100 per cent. This is often quoted as proof of the ingrained differences between the sexes. Except it's not true. These figures came from a Hewlett Packard internal report and the claim was later debunked in 2014 when an investigative journalist discovered there was no quantitative data to support the results. It was a masterclass in marketing, but it was not evidence of anything remotely scientific. That didn't stop people from believing it. A decade later and female athletes still refer to this report as an exemple of women underestimating their abilities. The same thing happens when you ask them why women can beat men at ultra distances. The longer the distance the more a race becomes about psychology rather than physiology, they respond. Women are more prepared. Women are better at multitasking. Women have more intuition. Women are more effective problem solvers. Women prioritise self-care and maintenance. Women have less ego. Women power through. These are the phrases that are bandied around. There are cases of exceptional women doing all of these things in this book, but is there actually any empirical evidence to back up these claims?

Female athletes will tell you that psychology plays a huge role in their advantage over males but when you dig deep, the science doesn't necessarily stand that up. There is no conclusive evidence that women and men measure differently when it comes to executive function. This common term in neuropsychology refers to the processes that enable us to plan, focus attention, remember, and juggle multiple tasks. These are all vital skills in endurance racing but there is nothing in the brain that sets the sexes apart. Results in multitasking tests are mixed and problem-solving studies have proved inconclusive. In fact, there are far more within sex differences than between sex differences, and lots of contradictory evidence. However, there is some evidence which demonstrates men are likely to overestimate abilities – such as their IQ, how quickly they can finish a race, or their physical fitness. The hypothesis is that this is driven by gender stereotypes. Conversely, women tend to underestimate their intelligence. The Hewlett Packard research may have been debunked, but a robust study conducted by the UK Government Equalities Office did find men were more willing to apply for a role than similarly qualified women. Men would apply for a job when they met 52.1 per cent of the qualifications, whereas women applied if they met 55.7 per cent. The small gender difference was explained by less qualified men's greater self-perceptions in meeting the overall requirements than similarly qualified women. Corrine Malcolm, a professional ultra runner and coach, has seen this play out time and again in sport. 'I've coached a number of co-ed running camps,' she said. 'On the first day people self-elect into groups. And every single time the men are overconfident and put themselves in the fastest, going the furthest group and the women put themselves in a lower group. We end up sending guys down to a gentler, easier group and sending women up and telling them they are capable.' In psychology, it appears nurture plays a bigger role than nature because of the societal limits placed on women.

As we might expect, the study of the mind is complex and at times contradictory. A limited number of studies point to testosterone as a catalyst for male impulsion, risk taking and hubris, whilst women with their lower levels of testosterone tend more towards humility and flexible decision making. But the research in this field leans heavily on laboratory tests, mostly focusing on academic achievement and child development. The one exception is a psychological study of participants in the 268-mile Montane Winter Spine Race between 2012 and 2018. The race psychologist, Fiona Beddoes-Jones, explored the resilience techniques of competitors during hundreds of hours of observation while working on the course. She observed that women adapted to the tough, cold and snowy conditions by being better prepared, very flexible and better at personal management, so they suffered fewer issues with feet and hypothermia. She cited the protective value of oestrogen, which in studies in mice has demonstrated that females problem-solve and cope better with stress than males. 'If you cut the oestrogen off for the female mice, they respond poorly. Similarly, if you give the male mice oestrogen, they become better at multitasking and coping with stress and problem solving. They become as good as the female mice.'

The observations from Beddoes-Jones's research give a snapshot of what is happening on the ground but unfortunately, they are far from conclusive. There is paltry research on sex difference and sports performance, so drawing parallels with existing research and correlating it to the hugely variable world of ultra-endurance sport is a giant leap to take. Then there is the problem of unpicking the social from the biological. There may be a strong belief that psychological differences set women apart from men but unpacking this from societal influences and normative gender roles is nigh on impossible.

If women do have an inherent ability to problem-solve and multitask more effectively than men, is this due to biological differences in their brain which are wired to make them more adept at child rearing? Or have they simply adopted these skills in order to successfully juggle modern day life where they are expected to be both mothers and breadwinners? If there is anecdotal evidence that women are more meticulous than men when it comes to ultra-race preparation, is this because of some fundamental brain function or because they have less race experience and less confidence because of social constraints? What we do know is this. Brain imagery indicates that the sexes operate differently, making it possible to spot a female or male brain from a scan. The differences are recognisable enough that neuroscientists at Stanford University can guess the sex of a brain with 90 per cent accuracy. We also know there are sex differences in how women and men behave and the jobs that they do. Much of this is due to testosterone levels. However, norms change and vary significantly between cultures. So, if the brains of women and men look different is this because of nature or nurture? Is it imposed by biology or society? Curiously, in the Stanford research, the area of the brain which looked different was the social part. So perhaps society plays the biggest role of all. This would support the recognised theory that throughout millennia the brains of both sexes have evolved, as women and men have behaved differently in response to their social groupings and the instinct to survive. Pinpointing psychological sex differences in sport is futile because there are no black and white answers, owing to the vast differences within the sexes, let alone between them. 'The unicorn doesn't exist because it's too crude,' explains UK sports psychologist David Collins. The view that men are from Mars and women from Venus is nonsense, he goes on, because fundamentally we are all from Earth 'so let's just get on with it.' He has a point. Before he contradicts it. 'That said, women's attention to detail is better than men's. Generally. Women's expectation management is better than men's. Generally. Women's distraction techniques are better than men's. Generally. Tolerance of failure is better than men's, generally. But that word 'generally' means that we're still talking about massive differences within the sexes.'

This is where it gets really interesting. Anecdotally, women and men observe psychological differences between the sexes all the time, but science tells us this doesn't exist in biology. Something is happening socially. Another example of nurture trumping nature. This is where the biopsychosocial approach becomes important to examine sport. Collins explains that human development is impacted by a range of intercepting biological, psychological and social factors. These three factors are interrelated and in the real world inseparable. He lays out a neat example of this. If you were coaching an athlete in a new skill, biologically the athlete's brain chemistry will affect their attention and memory. Their sleep the previous and following night will affect consolidation. Psychologically, their beliefs, motivations, skillset and emotional status will impact their engagement with the activity and coach. Socially, their social environment will influence the perceived value of the activity, the credibility/status and relationship with the coach, and the norms of the sport will influence their perception of the activity. Collins says: 'Women are often better prepared. All of us are different and that preparation is a psychosocially-conditioned characteristic.'

...

While science can't tell us if women are better at cognitive skills like preparation and problem solving, patriarchal society can give us an insight. The mental load is almost exclusively held by women in the home, and they have less time for leisure pursuits due to balancing work, caring commitments, and domestic chores (see Chapter 6). Their lives are made up of multitasking chores, planning ahead and problem solving on the fly. It's no surprise then that this social conditioning can give women the edge when it comes to endurance feats which rely heavily on non-physical skills. A perfect example of this is the Tandem Wow duo, Catherine Dixon and Rachael Marsden, who broke the outright record for cycling around the world on a tandem bicycle. Dixon and Marsden took 263 days to circumnavigate the globe, cycling 18,000 miles, reaching home just before the initial 2020 lockdown. They beat the previous men's world record by more than 17 days, cycling through storms, wildfires, monsoon rains and brutal headwinds. They crossed 25 countries, covering five continents, and burned up to 4,000 calories daily. Much of their success can be attributed to their fastidious preparation, along with their ability to cope under pressure.

At the age of four, Catherine Dixon loved nothing more than sneaking out of her home in Walton-on-Thames on the outskirts of London to ride her bike. 'My mother never drove a car so if I wanted to get anywhere I would just cycle. No one ever taught me how to ride a bike, I taught myself. I had a big family, and I would ride out of our close to the local library, around the library and back again, before anybody noticed I wasn't there. That was a four-mile trip, and I could do it before supper.' Riding her bike felt completely liberating, but

Dixon could never shake the feeling that one day she would just get on her bike and keep going and going. It took 50 years for her to realise this dream. At the age of 54 she quit her job as a CEO of Askham Bryan agricultural college near York, northern England, and paired up with a motor neurone nurse consultant, Rachel Marsden, then 55, who she met on an organised cycle from London to Paris, and decided it was time to ride the world. Four-year-old Dixon would finally be able to get on her bike and keep riding in one direction without turning back. Marsden, who ran as an elite athlete in the London Marathon during her youth, and competed while in the army, had turned to cycling in her forties following continual running injuries. Niggling away at the back of her mind was an around-the-world cycling challenge. But it wasn't until she met Dixon that the pieces fell into place. The duo soon realised that a tandem ride, on a bicycle made for two, would be the ultimate test of their abilities and the perfect chance to set an outright world record. They would become the fastest people to circumnavigate the globe on a tandem bicycle.

At first glance, the two women were an unlikely pairing. Dixon spoke with a friendly posh accent, her soft mousy bob framing her slender face. Marsden had a no-nonsense military demeanour, with tightly cropped hair and a stern voice. But as a team they complemented each other, and neither underestimated the task ahead. Riding a tandem might sound easier because you have two people pedalling one bicycle, but in reality, it is far more difficult than solo cycling. The bike is heavier and more clunky to turn. The riders need to cycle in sync with the person at the back, the stoker, navigating, whilst the pilot up front has sole responsibility for steering.

Breaking the women's world record would have been the obvious choice, given the challenge ahead, but for Dixon and Marsden this goal was too comfortably within reach. From the outset they set their sights on breaking the men's world record held since 2018 by two UK doctors, Lloyd Edward Collier and Louis Paul Snellgrove. The male riders had bought a ready-made tandem off the shelf, tested it for a short period of time and ended up with their entire journey littered with mechanical failures and makeshift repairs. Realising they needed to take a different approach to their male counterparts, the female duo knew success lay in the groundwork they did before setting off on their globetrotting adventure. They needed a custom-made bike that could handle epic endurance and they needed to test it. Having a tandem bicycle made to their specifications made all the difference. The steel frame, although heavier than carbon, meant it could be fixed by welding, anywhere in the world. Reinforced wheels meant the bike was able to endure the strain of 263 days riding, and a bespoke frame meant the bike was micro-adjusted to their exact body types, making cycling as comfortable as possible. And having 48 spokes meant there was less risk of breakage. While the doctors toiled with multiple broken spokes, the women didn't have a single spoke snag. Once the tandem was perfected, Tandem WOW as they became known, tested it with rides across the country and back-to-back days. This enabled them to iron out initial problems and adjust accordingly. In the beginning Dixon suffered an acutely painful burning sensation in her feet. A quick adjustment to her cleat instantly removed the affliction.

Even with their fastidious planning, scrutinising world maps and micro adjusting the bike, it was inevitable that nine months on the road would not be without its problems. Whether it was running out of hormone replacement therapy patches in Australia, being chased by vicious dogs in Greece, or fixing mechanical failures in the desert, Tandem WOW systematically and calmly dealt with each setback. Multitasking became their day-to-day reality, and they used multiple inventive strategies to cope. When the chain came off the bicycle, they simply kept pedalling and reattached it on the move. Self-care was also kept in check, despite juggling the daily challenge of navigating and cycling 80-100 miles a day and finding somewhere to camp for the night. 'We were put up by a couple in Australia who were following us and they were really surprised how un-smelly and nasty we were, because the guys had stayed with them previously, and were in a whole different state,' recalls Dixon. Although the science tells a different story she believes they had something the male duo did not. 'We got very good at multitasking, and I really think there is something in that. Men can be too rigid and too inflexible. If something doesn't work, then you try something else. Cat and I had a different sort of brain that worked in a different way to problem solve.' Marsden agrees, saying the key to their swift problem solving was their adaptability. "You can't be phased by what is happening on the ground. You have to be able to say 'we planned to do this today but actually it's not going to happen and that's OK".'

While there is limited evidence to suggest that women solve problems differently to men, there is some suggestion that they draw from a wider range of strategies. Much of the research is contradictory, but one insightful paper from the University of Hull, in northern England, published in the Journal of Sports Science, sheds light on what could be happening in sport. Researchers studied a sample of 749 undergraduate athletes aged 18 to 38 who competed at club to international level. They interrogated the athlete's response to stressors and found there was a significant difference. Males reported more stressors relating to injury and errors than females and were far more likely to implement blocking as a coping mechanism, meaning they tried to block out stressful thoughts. Women, by contrast, used more planning, attempts to change technique and greater communication to cope with stressors. While the men tried to ignore the problem, the women changed tactics to combat it. Marsden, the pilot, experienced this directly when she got nerve damage in her hands due to the vibration shuddering through the bike day after day. Rather than grit her teeth through the pain, she taped her hands and placed them on stress balls fixed to the handlebars to reduce the impact of the tremor.

Dealing with adversity under extreme conditions really came to the fore when Tandem WOW became stranded in Nullarbor National

Park in South Australia. The mechanism that tightened the timing chain, which connected the pilot to the stoker, became seized after being deluged with sand and grit. The chain came off making the bike unrideable. It was 1,700 miles to the next bike shop in Adelaide. Covered in flies and sand, with no shade in sight, they spent seven hours in 40-degrees heat trying to fix the bike. They were close to the Nullarbor desert, which is largely uninhabited except for a few lonely roadhouses. The choice was this: try to flag down a ride back to Perth and lose five days of riding or fix the problem and carry on. Eventually, with the use of a nail file in their wash bag they were able to file down a lump caused by stone damage and get the bike operational again. With the temporary fix in place, they dusted themselves down, got back on Alice the bike, and rode their way across the desert to the first bike shop in Adelaide. Their experience has many of the markings of a classic case study of women who prepared, multitasked and problem-solved in a manner we would expect of their sex. Sadly, the science is far more opaque and – because of the gender roles imposed on women – it is almost impossible to pick apart the biological from the societal. Mental myths are not borne out of studies in the lab but evolve into a constructed reality by the stereotypes placed on women. These sexist constraints mean women have so much more to prove, especially in an environment where they have little sense of belonging (see Chapter 6). It is no wonder then, that under certain circumstances women are willing to battle it out, to the bitter end.

16.
STICKING IT OUT

The kayak sludged through the thick stinking mud inch by inch. Inside the boat the sweaty teammates heaved and grunted as their paddles fought against the cow-poo-laden slush. Outside, standing waist-high in the muck, two more women pushed in silence. They were going to get to the checkpoint even if it took hours to cover the final few kilometres. Working as a team using the might of sheer doggedness they crept forward. They had been trekking via kayak, bike and foot for almost three days and it was time to put it all out there. The Australian adventure racers fiercely hoped no other team would attempt this relentless journey through the claggy mud, their refusal to give up acting as the ultimate trump card. It was time to play it. With half a kilometre to go team leader Kim Beckinsale decided to change tactics. It was time to wade through the head-high bullrushes, heaving the kayak and all their gear above them. It would have been far easier to ditch the boat and hike to the checkpoint, but the rules of this expedition stated the kayak must reach within five metres of the checkpoint. Slashing their way through the reeds dragging the vessel with their battered bodies they finally made it. On paper, the 15km paddle should have taken a couple of scenic hours but unbeknown to race organisers the estuary had been drained, leaving behind an oozing slurry of cattle waste.

The Mountain Designs Wild Women were the only team in the 2024 Legend Expedition Adventure Race to even attempt the mud crossing which took four hours of bloody-mindedness. Ninety minutes of this was spent dragging the kayak a mere 500 metres. They were able to dig deeper to achieve what at first seemed impossible, finding an inner strength in suffering. The male team who had been on their heels for the entirety of the event decided to take a time penalty instead of battling the sludge. This cost them first place position, while the women's determination to collect all 52 checkpoints no matter how tough the terrain, was awarded with a record-breaking outright win. Emitting a palpable stench of vomit, cow muck and salt-encrusted sweat as they crossed the finish line at Apollo Bay in south east Australia, they became the first all-female team to win an Adventure Race World Series expedition event, not just in Australia but internationally. This was a historic moment in adventure racing. It was the first time an all-women's team had won a major international race in 23 years of global competitions. The band of resilient women had raced non-stop for 450km navigating by map and compass, only occasionally snatching pockets of sleep. Whilst the course was open for six days, they finished in half the time in an impressive 73 hours and nine minutes. Like many adventure races, the course involved mountain and coastal trekking, mountain biking, plus ocean, river and lake kayaking. Led by Beckinsale, the quartet had an average age of 49, and 78 years of adventure racing experience between them. Despite their wealth of experience, the win itself was something of a controversy as only mixed-sex teams were allowed to participate as elites and qualify for the world championships.

Since the Raid Gauloises in New Zealand back in 1989, the sport had prioritised mixed-gender teams, meaning only those groupings were allowed to participate competitively. Adventure Racing World Series argues that teams of any gender mix can race and it is 'the only sport where men and women compete together on equal terms'. But here's the rub. A mixed team only has to feature one person of the opposite sex. As a result, many teams are made up of three men plus one 'token' woman who can be viewed as nothing more than a compulsory piece of equipment. An all-female or all-male team is not classified as premier and cannot qualify for the world championships. Despite their conclusive win, Wild Women were not eligible to compete at the next level. It appeared that the sport's ruling body had never considered that an all-female team might cross the line first. This caused an initial row for Beckinsale and her team when they were announced as the overall Legend winners, because technically they had won their category, but not the elite race. They were ineligible for the outright win because there was not a man on their team. The mixed team who came in 25 hours later won the spot at the world championships.

This gender disparity in the sport, which leans heavily in favour of men, was one of the reasons Beckinsale, a veteran adventurer, decided to form a different kind of team. The 56-year-old knew all about doing things 'the hard way' as this was the mantra she used in the playground while working as a high school PE teacher in Queensland, Australia. This was the woman who turned her back on a professional career in triathlon to become a teacher and coach, and who got into adventure racing not long after being hit by a car and fracturing her back. She was made of strong stuff but always thrived when working with others. Having raced in world-series-winning mixed teams for years she decided it was time to seek a new challenge. Realising that in all her adventure racing career she had rarely been given a map or the opportunity to navigate, she decided it was time to pay it forward and pass on her knowledge to other women, so they would continue racing long after she retired. The best way to do this was to set up a women's team, so that everyone had the opportunity to navigate and were not sidelined by men. While in mixed teams the navigator tended to be a fast man at the front setting the pace, whether they were the best map reader or not, in a women's team Beckinsale would navigate from the middle, recognising that the team worked as one. There was no pressure for individuals to prove they were the best. Joining Beckinsale in Wild Women were a sports entrepreneur, Alina McMaster, 55, a civil servant, Del Lloyd, 44, and a PE teacher, Cass Kimlin, 42.

Despite being the team leader, Beckinsale had to rely heavily on her companions at the beginning of the Legends race. Suffering from uncontrollable vomiting during the first day, her team rallied around her, deciding to take an unscheduled sleep to enable her to recover. 'I am not normally the person in the team suffering really badly. But I went from a high of smashing it mentally and physically to rock bottom. What was amazing was the way the team dealt with it. They weren't trying to drag me to a level I wasn't capable of. Instead they decided to stop and see if rest would help, even though it was the first night and we wouldn't normally stop,' recalls Beckinsale. Rallying around her, the team began by giving Beckinsale medication and stopping for 40 minutes to let it get into her system. Then they rummaged through her backpack for items to keep her warm, helping her to dress in a jacket, before covering her with a foil blanket. Once she was able to move, the next step was to spread her gear among them, because despite her tanned muscular physique the vomiting had made her too weak to carry the heavy kit. There was no way she was dropping out; this was just another problem to be solved. This resolve, not just to continue, but to plough onwards with no complaints, is seen time and again amongst female competitors. This mental resilience is all the stronger when a band of women work together. 'Those times when we had to deal with adversity, we were really cohesive', says Lloyd. 'Alina was seasick after three hours of kayaking on the sea. We noticed she hadn't eaten for four hours so we were feeding her jelly snake sweets, checking the pace was alright for her and making sure she had water. If we had big egos we would be really bothered about slowing down or stopping for Alina and Kim, but as a team you put all your energy together. There is always someone to buoy you up, or you are busy buoying someone else up. Working with women in adventure racing is really cool because there are no egos, no pretence, we're just all there to get through.'

Talking ten-to-the-dozen, the slightly framed Lloyd, one of the babies of the group at age 44, knows how vital communication is in adventure racing. The navigator is constantly giving verbal instructions on how far the next turning is, what the terrain will be like underfoot, and what landmarks to look out for. Team members constantly check in with one another to ensure they are all drinking and eating enough, the pace is manageable, and they are staying alert. There is hardly a moment's silence as they discuss each stage of the race on the fly, always trying to stay one step ahead of the next problem. Through a combination of communication, social support, empathy and respect this particular team were able to drag themselves through a series of sticky and sickly situations. Often, they used humour and laughter to bolster their spirits, singing songs or inventing news bulletins about their progress through the expedition. Beckinsale, who raced happily for years in mixed teams, believes there is something unique about how women pool together to develop inner strength. 'Women bring out the best in each other and communicate differently. If you are a female in a mixed team and you aren't pulling your weight allegedly, it's like 'what's wrong with you?' I don't think anyone means it to be that way but that's how it can sometimes come across as the difference between male and female. The way females react to the same situation is different. I don't know why that happens, but it just does,' says Beckinsale.

The tendency for females to tend and befriend in stressful situations may be one explanation for this variance in behaviour. While the human stress response has typically been characterised in social neuroscience as fight-or-flight for almost a century, most of this research has been conducted on males. In the early 2000s, a new bio-behavioural theory was put forward by researchers at the University of California. They proposed that the human female response to stress was not the fight-or-flight pattern seen predominantly in men but was instead characterised by tend-and-befriend. They surmised that female stress responses had selectively evolved to maximise the survival of self and offspring, by exhibiting behaviours that protected them from harm and affiliating with social groups to reduce risk. This may explain why ahead of the 2025 Montane Winter Spine Race a group of elite female athletes, including Sarah Perry (see Chapter 20), headed to the Pennine Way to train together. These women were all serious contenders, racing to win, but they were choosing to form a supportive community rather than a competitive one. This fits with the hypothesis of those Californian researchers who concluded that females create, maintain and utilise social groups, especially relations with other females, to manage stressful conditions. These tend-and-befriend patterns were thought to be oxytocin-mediated and moderated by sex hormones. But while the sex-linked neuroendocrine response to stress was biologically driven, the researchers hypothesised that the tend-and-befriend pattern was maintained by social and cultural roles. Once again, the unpicking of biology and sociology was a fruitless task with both sciences inextricably interwoven into human behaviour.

Whether nature or nurture, this female proclivity to lean markedly into social strategies when under immense pressure is a practice also observed in sports science. While male athletes prefer to use problem-focused coping strategies in response to stressors such as pain, injury, and criticism, females prefer emotion-focused coping in response to the same stressors. Several studies have found support for the notion that females are more likely to use social support to cope with stressors while men use greater suppression techniques. Using the social support of their team, Wild Women utilised compassion and nurturing to their advantage when faced with adversity. Whether it was caring for a sick teammate or communicating progress as they inched through the gruelling mud, they chose expression over suppression.

This combination of mental toughness and self-compassion is defined as the Zipper Effect in an influential 2019 study published in the journal Psychology of Sport and Exercise. The researchers interviewed elite Canadian women athletes about their perceived and experienced mental toughness and self-compassion, and their compatibility in the pursuit of athletic success and stress management. Mental toughness enables athletes to persevere through difficult situations to achieve their goals and has long been established as a positive psychological process for managing the stress of high-performance demands. Mentally tough athletes tend to cope more effectively with stressors and report higher levels of perceived control and lower levels of distress and anxiety. Self-compassion may on face value appear to be the antithesis of toughness, but the ability to be kind and non-judgmental towards oneself when faced with pain, suffering and failure is a critical coping resource. It enables athletes to regulate emotion by buffering against the negative effects of self-judgement and to be able to move forward after setbacks with a positive perspective. Nevertheless, there is a balance to be struck. Too much mental toughness can result in pushing through pain and injury, and not seeking timely medical support. Silencing emotional difficulty, under the guise of toughness, is a typically masculine trait which, as seen in the previous chapter, can lead to unrealistic goals and poorer results. The best outcome is found when mental toughness and self-compassion are in harmonious balance, creating the optimal mindset for the pursuit of athletic success.

While the Wild Women had one another to rely on for compassion and motivation, for the lone athlete this isn't an option. Self-care becomes crucial in the latter stages of an ultra-endurance event, when rest, fuel, hydration and clothing become as important as movement. Jasmin Paris was acutely aware of this when temperatures plummeted during her record-breaking Spine Race (see Chapter 1) and she layered up with every piece of clothing she was carrying. Chasing her down, Eugeni Roselló Solé opted for less gear to lighten his load and increase his speed, which proved a dire mistake. He was rescued from the course suffering from hypothermia with less than four miles to go. As the psychologist Fiona Beddoes-Jones observed across six years of the 268-mile race, women were better at self-management and suffered fewer issues with the cold weather and had far fewer foot problems (see Chapter 15). Sabrina Verjee who meticulously planned her Wainwrights record (Chapter 14) knew how important fuelling was to maintain her steady pace. At the sharp end of an ultra race, speed and strength are no longer the controlling factors. Self-preservation and mental resilience are. Josephine Perry, a sports psychologist who works with elite and amateur athletes, says nutrition is an essential component of ultra marathons, and not looking after your body's energy requirements can be disastrous. Correctly and continuously fuelling your body will also fuel your brain, increasing the chances of good decision making and mental strength. She explains: 'Your brain is five per cent of your body weight, but it uses 20 per cent of the energy that you put into your body. I find women are better at maintaining their fuel link so they can stay in the right mindset for completion. More men will respond to the feelings within the body and stop eating when they feel really nauseous and as a result under-fuel their brain. That means a DNF or a performance they weren't hoping for.'

Undoubtedly, nutrition is critical when it comes to self care but it extends far beyond this. All the small things matter when you are active for hours, or days, on end. Everything from applying suncream, to changing socks, to dunking a hat in ice-cold water, can make a record-breaking difference.

Speed does not triumph self care, as Eleanor Baverstock, a club runner, discovered when she won an inaugural 50-mile race outright. The lean but muscular marathon runner, who always runs with a huge smile on her face, comfortably won the Epping Forest Ultra, in the south east of England, at the age of 30. Racking up 100 miles of running most weeks, the striking brunette trains as hard as her male counterparts, but in this ultra-marathon race that didn't give her the edge. While at the time her fastest marathon was a remarkable 2:52:48, she was up against sub-2:30 marathoners at the woodland start line. It was a sultry and humid September day, and temperatures peaked at 28 degrees Celsius over the course of the 10 laps. Racing through forest paths, the runners navigated 100 metres of elevation on each loop, dodging long-horn cows, muntjac and fallow deer.

For the first four laps, a male runner took the lead chased down by a posse from Orion Harriers including three men and Baverstock. The lead changed hands numerous times as the race progressed, and the heat and humidity took its toll. The man leading the race for the first half wilted away, while Baverstock continued to gain strength, finishing first in 7:15:26. Deliberately playing the long game Baverstock prioritised self-care and ensured she stayed on top of fluid and fuel, as the temperatures soared on an unusually hot autumnal day. 'It really shows the example of us females being a bit more strategic in our race, and men being quite happy to go off flying and then blow up spectacularly,' Baverstock says. 'I was around fifth place for the first few laps. I had some gut problems so I knew I had to manage that so I could continue with the rest of the race. If I needed to go to the toilet, I did. If I wanted to stay a bit longer at the aid station I did. I would pick my snack up from the aid station and walk out. The guys were very much keep running, keep going. By halfway through the race I was passing some of the guys and asking them if they were OK. They hadn't been thinking about their fuelling strategy, they hadn't been thinking about getting enough fluid and salts in. Some of the guys had only eaten one gel. They were starting to struggle and I took the lead on lap six and extended it until the end of the race.' For Baverstock, running hundreds of miles a month was not adequate training. She also practised fuelling, hydration, applying sun cream and running in all weather conditions so she knew how to look after herself when things got tough.

...

The capacity for resilience underpinned by self-care can level the playing field between the sexes in ultra sport, tipping it in favour of those women who have the race – and life – experience to know when to push, and when to hold back. This experience comes through years of racing and the passage of time as competitors become more adept at reading their bodies and managing the problems ultra endurance throws at them.

17.

OLDER AND FASTER

She couldn't breathe. The icy air lodged in her throat as a wave of devastation washed through her trembling body. 'I can't cry' she told herself, 'my tears will freeze'. Alone in a barren icy wilderness with nothing but whiteness stretched out before her, Mimi Anderson had to keep moving. Her father was dead. He was more than 2,000 miles away, but at that moment she knew he was gone. The final 120 frozen miles would push her physical and mental resilience to the absolute limit but she was determined to finish. This was for Dad.

The extraordinary journey had begun just days earlier as Anderson, age 44, set out to win the inaugural Arctic 6633-foot race. Pulling a sled with all her supplies she had eight days to cover 352 miles non-stop across the harshest landscape of northern Canada. Temperatures dropped to -40 degrees Celsius, with the biting wind making it feel like an inextricable -70. Anderson was taking 'me time' to the extreme. This was the blonde-bobbed British mother-of-three who loved to snuggle up in front of the fire at her Kent home, sipping white wine from a lipstick-stained glass. This was the woman who spent two decades battling anorexia and only started running because she wanted slim legs. This was the little girl who suffered horrific abuse from her childhood nanny, who thrust her finger in an exposed light socket and dragged her downstairs by the feet. This was the powerless seven-year-old who stood and watched as her younger sister fell into a frozen Norwegian lake after being forced onto the ice by their cruel nanny. This was the woman, past the age of sporting peak performance, who was unwavering in her belief that she would win this race. As counterintuitive as it sounds, Anderson knew that in ultra-endurance racing, competitors often got stronger with age – in direct contrast to other sports. What was driving this age enigma? Was it physiology, psychology or society?

...

Anderson's first melee with running occurred when she took to the treadmill at the age of 36. As a stay-at-home mum going to the gym offered a break from parenting and an opportunity to socialise with others. By this point she had a relatively healthy relationship with food but unresolved issues with body image, making her strive for the 'perfect' legs. Running was a means to tone her limbs, rather than to lose weight and she set herself the challenge of running a mile. This was her first ever running target and a momentous occasion when she finally achieved it. Encouraged to try running outside by gym buddies, Anderson soon discovered she had a knack for endurance. No longer obsessed with how her legs looked, she saw them as a tool to aid her running performance and she wanted them to feel as strong as possible. Regaining confidence in her muscular body, she ensured she fuelled herself properly and signed up for her first half marathon. Buzzing from the race, she took a leap of faith signing up with female friends for the Marathon des Sables, a 250km seven-day race in the Sahara Desert. Being away from her children for 12 days was a new experience – one which she was criticised for, particularly when her son Ruaraidh was hospitalised the day before she flew out. A freak accident with a classroom door had left him with the handle embedded in his arm. Anderson rushed him to hospital for stitches and, as her bandaged child lay in recovery, she realised the impossible choice ahead. Stay at her son's bedside or stick to the plan and leave. The maternal instinct screamed at her to stay but the desire to be a runner, a role model, a trailblazer and an inspiration to her children told her to go. Reassured by doctors that Ruaraidh would make a full recovery (he did) and persuaded by her husband Tim that she couldn't let all her training and hard work go to waste, she packed her bags and headed for Morocco.

Despite the demanding conditions and mum guilt, the Marathon des Sables was the turning point in her running career. Over the next decade, Anderson spent her forties building up podium positions. While it may have seemed like she was bucking the peak performance trend, in the world of ultra running late bloomers like Anderson remain the norm rather than the exception. Women in particular tend to start racing later in life, often post-children, enabling them to draw on decades of resilience and life experience, giving them a few years' edge over men. This phenomenon baffles Professor Hans Degens, an expert on muscle physiology who has spent his life studying age-related changes in skeletal muscle morphology. Over the past four decades his work has taken him from the Netherlands to the UK, USA, Sweden, and back to the UK again, resulting in 200 scientific journal publications. The avid cyclist and herpetologist (the study of amphibians and reptiles) regales his youthful days when he was content to cycle 250km in a day, pitch up a tent and then repeat it all again the following morning. Now in his sixties he is exhausted after a 12km ride and seeks out home comforts rather than outdoor adventures. He says this is due to the natural deterioration of the body during the ageing process rather than a lack of fitness. His dinner party chat is now filled with tales of aching joints and tired muscles as friends compare notes on their declining athleticism. This may be frustrating for Degens but it simply reflects all of his research.

The human body begins breaking down around the age of 30 with a steady drop in physical strength and agility, before this is ramped up several gears from age 70 onwards, accelerating rapidly in our final decades. There is just a small window when humans are at their physical peak. Studies across a huge variety of speed and endurance sports reveal that, physiologically speaking, peak performance occurs between the ages of 24 and 28. Once we enter our fourth decade, there is no denying the progressive loss of muscle mass which decreases both our power generating capacity and flexibility. In the cardiovascular system, there is a steady decline in stroke volume and cardiac output, contributing to decreasing performance as our hearts become more inefficient at pumping blood. We do not get better at endurance with age. Slow and fast-twitch fibres decline. Lactate threshold reduces. Everything is physically harder. Yet this appears to contradict the evidence coming out of the ultra-endurance field where time and again older athletes win world-class races and set mind-boggling records. Recreational athletes also peak later.

Scribbling rudimentary graphs on a piece of scrap paper, Degens explains how sedentary people who come to exercise later in life can still make 30 per cent performance gains. There is one higher performance line for athletes and a lower performance line for the control group. But it is possible to bridge this gap through training. Both lines curve downwards from the age of 28 so even with 30 per cent gains an elite athlete of age 40 will never be as physiologically strong as their elite 28-year-old rival. What is happening in ultra sport is something else. Athletes are coming to the sport later in life but there are also huge psychological elements at play. Maybe this is why an ageing Julius Caesar was able to fight alongside his young soldiers during the Gallic Wars 2,000 years ago, muses Degens. He was able to endure the hardship of those decades younger than him because of something far less tangible or measurable than physicality. Caesar had grit. This determination, which manifests itself in the mind, rather than the body, is replicated in today's older endurance athletes. Ultra-race results back this up. Numerous scientific studies have shown the age of peak performance increases with distance, and the gap between women and men narrows, too. Females keep peaking well into their fifties while men tend to reach the top of their ultra game in their late forties. The historic 56-mile (89km) Comrades race in South Africa is a case in point. In this ultra road race women reach their best performance six years later than men.

The evidence keeps mounting up. A comprehensive study of the age of peak running speed from 1969 to 2012 examined the results of 205,577 finishes (4,254 women and 201,323 men) in distances from 50km to 1,000km. The results were a welcome surprise for older athletes wanting to run further. The best female 1,000km ultra marathoners were seven years older than the best female 100km runners. At all distances, peak performance occurred in women's thirties right the way through to their mid-fifties. This is strikingly different to marathon and Olympic performance, where the peak is reached in the mid to late twenties.

Present data confirms that high-level performances in 100km ultra marathons can be achieved at a higher age than marathon distance, especially for women. Similar patterns are found across ultra triathlon, cycling and swimming, where women in their thirties all the way up to their late forties perform better than their youthful competitors in Ironman distances, 720km cycles, and 12-hour swims. So, it's no surprise then that Anderson was racking up podium positions well into her late forties. She excelled at the most extreme races, whether it was running 100 miles in the Himalayas, 155 miles across the blazing Kalahari Desert or a particularly unpleasant 120-mile self-sufficiency race in Libya. And she was doing all of this whilst dealing with something men don't even have to consider. Menstruation. 'I went to the Libya race and my period wasn't due to start until after I got back and it started on race day. Now you're in 50-degree heat with a period and you are running 120 miles and you can't wash, you can't shower. It was absolutely disgusting but I had to get on with it. I hadn't got a choice,' she recalls matter-of-factly.

Things weren't about to get any easier for Anderson. Having conquered the soaring temperatures of several desert ultras, she wanted to test her limits by dropping way below zero. The decision to leave for the Arctic challenge was particularly wrenching as her father was diagnosed with terminal bladder cancer just three weeks before the race day. But he insisted she continue with the race, saying it would distract him from the pain. Tracking her progress online from his hospital bed, Anderson's father was awash with pride. Knowing he was watching, Anderson vowed to give it everything she had and told her husband she was going to win. Despite her determination to beat the men, she refused to behave like 'one of the lads' and would often turn up to ultra marathons dressed in her signature pink, wearing a skirt and make-up. At the ice trucker hotel, the night before the Arctic 6633 a band of drunken truckers were in disbelief that Anderson, a petite 40-something woman, was planning to do such a crazy event. They weren't the only men with their noses out of joint, as Anderson soon discovered in the early stages of the race. 'I remember there was a guy and he had a thing about being beaten by women. I don't think he liked me very much. It was extraordinary to watch as he was chasing me. I remember thinking: "I don't know why you're doing that? We're 20 miles into the race, you've got 352 miles to cover". So, I just let him go. I had my plan and I stuck to it. I then overtook him at about 45 miles as he was sleeping, and I never saw him again.' She was so far ahead that Anderson barely saw a single soul during the whole race, only coming into contact with humans at the sparsely spread-out checkpoints. Crossing the finish line in 145 hours and 23 minutes, Anderson was a phenomenal 24 hours ahead of the next competitor, much to the bemusement of the local truckers. Her course record still stands today.

Despite edging closer to her 50th birthday, Anderson was only just getting into her stride. Only now she didn't have to contend with periods, she was battling the menopause instead. When her periods stopped, Anderson felt a 'hallelujah' moment, but this was swiftly replaced by a tsunami of night sweats, aching limbs and lethargy. 'It was a nightmare, and I didn't really understand it because we didn't talk about it then,' Anderson says. 'It was just horrible. I felt really lethargic and yet nothing had changed. My bones ached a lot in my legs. I found running ultras really hard sometimes. And there wasn't really information out there because they tend to do all testing on male rather than female athletes.' Now on 'the other side' in her sixties she puts her outstanding performances down to experience, knowledge and resilience which is something she believes develops with age, giving older ultra-endurance athletes the edge. 'It all comes from experience. I got better as I got older and I felt stronger. Recovery in my fifties took slightly longer but I had years of experience behind me. When you run 100 miles even if you're an experienced runner it's gonna hurt you regardless of where you come from, but I think if you're more experienced, you know how to handle it slightly better because it's not just the physical side. There's also the mental side as well.'

This goes some way towards explaining how in 2008, aged 46, Anderson set an astonishing female world record. She ran 840 miles from John O'Groats, the most northerly point in mainland Britain to the southern tip of the country called Land's End. The records kept coming. Going back to her gym roots, she set a female world record covering 403.81 miles on a treadmill in seven days, aged 48. And then there were the string of doubles, running Comrades 56-mile South African race twice (112 miles), and setting a female course record for the Badwater 135-mile (170 miles) and Grand Union Canal 145-mile (190 miles) doubles. It seemed that everywhere Anderson ran, she set a world record. By now a grandmother, Anderson recorded the fastest crossing on foot across Ireland in 2012, age 50 (before Sophie Power set a new record in 2024, see Chapter 18), and less than 12 months later became the first person to complete a double Grand Union Canal race, totalling 290 miles from London to Birmingham and back again. She followed this up, aged 52, by becoming the only person to finish the 2014 Cyprus Ultra, setting yet another course record on the non-stop 135-mile route. The following year she became the first female to complete a double Spartathlon, running the 156-mile course in just 35 hours and seven minutes, before running back to the start again. Even with numerous records to her name Anderson still felt she was treated differently to her male competitors. She recalls her frustration at the final checkpoint of the Cyprus Ultra she won outright. 'I remember on the last lap I was literally the last person standing and the organiser at the checkpoint came up to me and said Mimi you can sit down, you can have a rest, you can have a sleep, you've got loads of time. I said: "This is a race, would you say this to a man? No, you would say come on you can do this, you can go and get the record." I found that very odd.'

The disbelief that an older woman was capable of such incredible endurance feats continued into her 2017 world record attempt across America. Fifty-five-year-old Anderson was followed by a man determined to prove she was cheating. He drove dangerously close to her through the state of Kansas before her crew eventually had to call the police. Anderson, who ran 55 miles a day on average, completed a phenomenal 2,217 miles in 40 days before injury forced her to retire short of her 2,870-mile target. A scan revealed bone oedema, which was causing her agonising pain. The cartilage had worn away so severely there was nothing but bone rubbing on bone on the side of her knee. Anderson was prepared to run through the pain but did not want to risk long-term damage preventing her from ever running again, so reluctantly stopped less than 600 miles from her target. Many would have retired from endurance at this point but resolute as ever to test her capacity for endurance she simply switched to cycling. At the age of 61 this culminated in a 4,400km ride from Turin in Italy to North Cape, Norway, across 10 countries in under three weeks. Something a similarly aged Degens could only dream of.

···

Anderson's athletic journey through the decades is testament to the power of psychology over physiology in ultra distances. It's also a reminder of how many women come to the sport later in life when they are desperate to carve out time for themselves outside of career pressures and family caring duties. They may be older, but they are wiser. Their time is more precious, so they take a meticulous approach to training. This culminates in older women entering ultra races with a wealth of life experience, careful preparation and swathes of determination which over gruellingly long distances counts for far more than male speed. Older women have learned how their bodies react to stress, exercise, fuelling and sleep deprivation. They know how to train and how to adapt. Decades of life experience through puberty, adulthood, motherhood and menopause has taught them how to understand the nuances of the female body, what it requires, and where its strength lies. Unfortunately, the ultra landscape is not operated by women, meaning these distinctions are lost in gender translation. In an environment where the male lens prevails the biggest hurdle to overcome is female knowledge deficit. Until this void is filled, women will continue to face unnecessary barriers to entry.

18.
BARRIERS TO ENTRY

The body lay strewn on the floor, scattered bottles surrounding it. Intermittent groans disrupted the silence as the feeding frenzy ensued. Emaciated bodies continued streaming through the doors, stumbling over discarded clothes and shoes. Amid the chaos, a woman with short dark curls sat staring at her three-month-old baby. She had been running sleepless through the night scaling the Alps on her 105-mile journey. While she breastfed her baby, simultaneously expressing milk from her second exposed breast, a photographer approached her. Sophie Power was a little under halfway through the Ultra-Trail du Mont-Blanc (UTMB) and was stopping to feed herself and her son Cormac at an aid station near the Italian ski resort of Courmayeur. The exhausted male runner lay next to her chair, feet raised in the air attempting to relieve the pressure of his aching limbs. But Power, who had become accustomed to sleep deprivation in the three months prior to the race, was feeling strong. Her goal at this checkpoint was to simply keep her milk supply going. She had been trying to hand express on the trails, ducking behind trees to relieve her painful breasts as they gradually became engorged with milk. Cormac usually fed every couple of hours, but it had been 16 since mother and son had united. This was her first opportunity to sit down and feed her child.

...

What happened next triggered a seismic debate about motherhood. Within days the image of Power breastfeeding had gone global. The amateur runner, who did not have an Instagram account at the time, was not prepared for the subsequent attention she received on social media. The overwhelmingly positive response to the photo was a springboard for Power to open the discussion on motherhood and identity. 'We shouldn't have to lose who we were before we were mothers,' argues Power. 'There is this huge mother's guilt that all the time you need to be 100 per cent focused on your baby. But for me personally I need to be physically fit, and to have those mental health breaks, to be a good mum. Women really struggle to be able to say that.' The image was a visceral reminder that mothers were as strong, capable, and enduring as men, and equally deserved a place on the start line. But it also highlighted the woefully inadequate pregnancy deferral policies of races and how women's circumstances were not being considered. As this book has demonstrated time and again, sexual discrimination is rife in ultra-endurance sports. From the unequal coverage (Chapter 5), to the gaping deficit in research (Chapter 8), through to the lack of women on the starting line (Chapter 6). From the outset, women are at a disadvantage.

...

Power was only in the race because unlike a man, she had no option of deferring. To enter the highly competitive UTMB, Power needed to earn points by running other ultras within a set timeframe. She had secured a place at the 2014 UTMB but had to give it up because she was six months' pregnant with her first son, Donnacha. While injured athletes were able to defer their place, at the time UTMB did not allow women to defer if they became pregnant. In 2018, having landed another place, Power was caught out once more, as her due date was just three months before the race starting date. She faced a dilemma: run the race or spend years amassing points once more. Once the UTMB photo of Power went viral she was contacted by embarrassed male race directors at other events who admitted they had never thought about their pregnancy policy. At the same time Power was receiving messages from women frustrated with barriers to ultra participation. She began working with race companies to develop fair pregnancy deferral policies and, in 2020, became a board trustee of Women in Sport. It wasn't long before she realised deferral policies were just the tip of the iceberg. The messages from women kept pouring in. They felt unseen and excluded from the world of ultra endurance. Power decided she could no longer stand on the sidelines, acting as a consultant to others. She needed to capitalise on that photograph and take decisive action. She wanted to give all those unheard women a voice. She wanted to create a racing environment where women felt comfortable, welcome, and confident.

The feeling of imposter syndrome resonated with Power. Like many women she came to running later in life, picking up the pace when she had children in her thirties. It became an important mechanism for creating physical and mental space during early motherhood. As the CEO of environmental tech company Airlabs, juggling work and family life was demanding, but running enabled her to switch off and unload. Hitting the oak-tree-strewn Surrey Hills in southeast England, Power found solitude on the clay trails. Like so many other women she had never seen herself as a sporty girl. She vividly remembers coming second to last in the school mile at the impressionable age of 14. In sixth form, she would sneak off to eat pizza and watch the Australian soap opera Neighbours at her mate's nearby house whilst the rest of the year did cross country. Jogging the short distance back to the school gates an hour later, she desperately tried to look tired.

Little did she know that two decades later she would be representing Great Britain in the 24-Hour World Championships in Taiwan.

The experience of UTMB, and the global reaction from disenfranchised women, solidified her view that endurance events were inadvertently creating sex-based barriers. Realising race directors, the vast majority of whom were men, needed support to adjust their male lens, she set up SheRACES in the UK in 2022. The non-profit organisation exists to level the starting line and remove barriers to entry which put women off. While Power recognises some of the barriers are societal, she strongly believes many are down to the events themselves. 'They don't realise they're putting these barriers in place,' Power says. 'But typically, if we look at the average race director, it's a middle-aged white man. We would significantly increase the amount of women on our start lines if races were designed through a female lens. If you open a race website the homepage is a picture of the start line and it's white skinny men.' SheRACES aims to drive positive change and increase female participation in running, triathlon and cycling events, particularly over longer distances. Viewing races through a female perspective, SheRACES recognises achieving equality in sport is not about treating women the same as men, because the barriers to participation are different. Gathering quantitative and qualitative data on running event barriers for women, SheRACES uncovered a multitude of challenges, which intensify the longer the distance. From logistical concerns about changing rooms, toilet facilities and cut-off times, to feeling excluded owing to male-fitting T-shirts, unequal coverage of women's and men's competition, and unequal prize money. Shockingly some 80 per cent of women had been given a male-fit T-shirt at the end of a race. Women clearly wanted something to change. In the survey, 88 per cent said they would be more likely to enter events committed to equitable and inclusive treatment for women. They were not asking for dramatic changes, a simple adjustment to a race cut-off time might make all the difference. A UK fell race allowing slower competitors to start an hour earlier doubled participation amongst women over 50 years, explains Power.

Women also needed vicarious role models. They needed to see women like them taking part in endurance events. Diverse imagery on websites and social media featuring people of all ages, abilities, sexes, sizes and ethnicities would sell the message 'this is a space for everyone'. Information was also vital to accessibility and women wanted to learn about the logistics of a race beforehand rather than be bamboozled by the obfuscation of ultra, with men as the gatekeepers. Practical information to aid race preparation was cited as a pivotal enabler by 60 per cent of women who spoke to SheRACES. Power says: 'We want to know how that's going to work for us. Where's the start? How do we get there? How do we make sure we can get home at night? What are the cut-offs? What kit do we need? What's the terrain like? Really visualising that day to make us believe that we can do it. And that's not provided on most websites.' Straight forward practical information didn't seem too much to ask for. Details on whether toilet facilities and sanitary products were provided could quickly ease a woman's concerns about entering a race and how they needed to prepare. Equipping checkpoints with hand sanitiser, wet wipes and sanitary bins was a quick, simple solution to aid hygiene during a woman's period. Yet this was never a consideration for many endurance races. Women were just expected to muddle through (see Chapter 17).

Safety concerns were also identified as a huge barrier for women, something that rarely concerns men. Wherever you turn in the world, women feel unsafe when running or have experienced some form of harassment. In a survey of 9,000 runners from nine countries, 92 per cent of women reported feeling concerned for their safety when running, with half afraid of being physically attacked compared to 28 per cent of men. The 2023 Adidas survey revealed 38 per cent of women had experienced verbal harassment while running. Over half had received sexist comments or unwanted attention. When Threshold

Sport ultra series surveyed 600 of its female participants, they found safety was the number one concern, with a third of women believing it was the biggest barrier to taking part. Safety is an enormous concern. It cannot be denied that sexual harassment on the roads and trails remains a significant issue for many women. A study of 1,500 trail and ultra runners published in the journal Social Sciences found incidents of catcalls, spanking, flashing, unwanted verbal advances, stalking, forced sexual acts and rape, were substantially higher among females. Seventy per cent of women reported incidents of sexual harassment and assault whilst running, compared to just 17 per cent of men. It is not uncommon for elite female athletes to be physically 'pushed out of the way' by men on a course or to feel threatened by a male competitor running closely behind them in the dark. 'The need to feel safe should never be underestimated by a race organiser. But we know that for many men it is difficult to understand,' says Power.

Cycling is even more extreme. In some ultra-cycling races participants are not allowed to stop and help one another without fear of being disqualified. Then there is the language used to frame these events, which are more often than not described as extreme, brutal or tough. The aggressive and macho vocabulary used in promotional race material, often overstates the achievability of a challenge, and deters women. The ultra runner Jasmin Paris, winner of the Spine Race (see Chapter 1), says: 'I think part of the problem is they will say it's the most brutal race in the world. All the words they use are extreme: most brutal and toughest. I think it's more likely to attract men. And these are hard races but I have no doubt that many more women would be completely fine. It's just knowing that they can do it, that's the problem.' Changing the language of race promotion is one easy barrier to remove, says the sports commentator Corrine Malcolm. 'Having it explained in a way where it's approachable, and it's not designed to be 'this is the hardest thing you're ever going to do' would be a positive change. We don't all need to be Navy Seals to circumnavigate a large mountain range.' Many ultra races are described as 'the biggest, baddest, toughest and really hard to finish' says Power. 'But when organisers describe a race rather than describing what will stop someone, they should turn it on its head and explain what pace they need to do in order to complete the race.' Although taking part in an ultra race is undoubtedly a huge undertaking, it is not an impossible one. But this less captivating truth is not the message conveyed by many race companies. They focus on the brutality of the event rather than the generous cut-off times and extensive support crews, which make the race accessible.

...

By pointing out to companies that they are potentially deterring huge swathes of the running community, organisations like SheRACES in the UK and Trail Sisters in the US are ushering in change. Gradually, their guidelines are being integrated by more race companies and a shift is happening. Pregnancy deferral policies are now in place at UTMB, Western States 100 and Hardrock 100 thanks to the work of these advocacy groups. Race companies are waking up to the desperate need for equality, as their policies and procedures are being called out. A few races are even running away from the norm. The Tarawera 100k race in New Zealand, one of the UTMB world series events, has 49 per cent female participation, as do several other Kiwi ultras. That's no surprise when their website homepages teem with the smiling faces of female trail runners. Some races are going as far as implementing 50:50 quotas, so once 50 per cent of male spaces are filled, they only allow female participants to enter. The High Lonesome 100 in Colorado, USA run by a husband-and-wife duo, is entered via a 50:50 female-male split lottery. The 500km Dead Ends & Cake self-supported bike packing race in Switzerland also draws participants in a 50:50 gender split via a lottery. The bucket list multi-day foot race Marathon Des Sables introduced single-sex tents, toilets and changing areas in 2024. Meanwhile in 2024, Threshold Trail

Series in the UK launched its Ultra 50:50 initiative. The ultra-running event company has achieved a higher-than-average proportion of female athletes since 2013 but pledged to go one step further to achieve 50 per cent participation. The campaign endeavoured to achieve gender parity and 'set new industry standards to inspire, empower and enable women to take part in events at the toughest end of the running distance spectrum'. The company worked with SheRACES to understand the barriers to participation and is working with female athletes to tackle representation, training, event access, safety, menstrual health and menopause, with a view to making women equally visible on the start line. This was followed by the Trailblazers Campaign in 2025 which is supporting 500 women to train for their first ultra marathon.

More races are introducing female-only recces, like 13 Valleys in the Lake District, UK, and it is more common to see female-only toilets at the start line of an endurance event. But there is still pushback. When Pen Llyn Ultra race series in Wales launched a female-only 50k event with no cut-off time and women's T-shirts at the finish line, they faced heavy criticism. The sold-out She Ultra event which attracted 500 women was accused of being regressive and exclusionary. The ultra-running world is a welcoming one, men on social media cried, so why do women need a no-male zone? Not all women need, or want, this type of event. However, the popularity of the inaugural race demonstrated that some women really did want a more comfortable space to try something new and difficult. Three-quarters of women at the 2024 She Ultra start line said they had been put off entering races by cut-offs. Most of the women had never run an ultra before (70 per cent) and 80 per cent strongly desired a female-only space. Even an experienced ultra runner like Power, who recounts being shoved off the trail by men during mixed races, felt safer on the She Ultra starting line. 'The race was special in so many ways – from the personal space on the start line – it felt very weird not to be crushed – to the abundance of toilets, female volunteers and just that atmosphere where I felt I could truly drop my guard.' It sent a clear message. Mixed-sex events still need to remove many barriers if female participation is to increase.

On that single day in May, 350 women in North Wales did something they had never attempted before. They ran an ultra marathon. By creating an environment in which they felt a sense of belonging, safety and possibility, they were able to challenge themselves and begin to explore what the female body is capable of. Something which Power strives to do year-on-year. Whilst she ran continuous loops for 24 hours around Taipei City, the capital of Taiwan, in early December 2023, her mind started plotting her next adventure. What if running non-stop for 24 hours was not her limit? What if she could take on a more extreme challenge to unite women around a cause and demonstrate what a mother of three young children could accomplish? By the end of the race, where she placed first British woman (19th female overall, running 227km), she had made her decision.

She would follow in the literal footsteps of her role model Mimi Anderson (see Chapter 17), another mother-of-three, and attempt a world record. With just five months to go, she began planning and training for the fastest crossing of Ireland on foot. This wasn't an arbitrary Guinness World Record attempt, it was deeply rooted in Power's family, and symbolised how motherhood could facilitate rather than limit a woman's potential. With an Irish husband, Power longed for her children to have a deeper connection to the country and experience an Irish adventure. It was immediately obvious to her that the best time to tackle the 347-mile challenge was during the school half-term holiday. That way Donnacha, nine, Cormac, six, and Saoirse, three, could be heavily involved. 'It was far more than about me doing the run. It was about the country, my kids and women setting challenges. I thought what an amazing thing for the boys to see Ireland and go through the whole country with me. And Saoirse would get to spend some time with her grandparents. I think in my head, the fact that I was just dropping her off (in southern Ireland), driving north, and running back to her, was just a very powerful imagery that I knew I could centre myself on and push really hard to do that,' explains Power.

Coining her endeavour Challenge You, Power used her large social media following to become a vicarious role model. She called on women to find their 'why' and set themselves a challenge with the support of their family and friends. 'We usually set limits on ourselves from the age of five years old. We don't think we're as good as boys at sport. As we get older and have children, we don't take that time for ourselves. I think there's huge power in setting a challenge and completing something that's outside our normal comfort zone. It could be running to the nearest town where your friend lives or cycling to work for the first time. It could be anything but needs to be something that's meaningful to you.' What struck Power most during the arduous journey were the women who came out to run with her, who were inspired to set their own challenges. 'They said, I get this. I have not thought about myself for years and I want to do something that is different because it's good for my mental and physical health. I didn't realise how strongly the message would resonate, especially with slightly older women.'

Taking on the dual responsibility of achieving a personal challenge whilst trying to embody a public symbol was Power's toughest trial to date. She began her epic journey in torrential rain and finished three days, 12 hours and eight minutes later under the blazing sun, at times close to collapsing from heat exhaustion. She knocked three and a half hours off the world record (there is no Guinness World Record for a man) at the age of 41, with her two older children crewing from a motorhome. As she arrived in Mizen Head, her left knee painfully swollen owing to the steep camber on the roads, three-year-old Saoirse asked mummy why she was crying. 'Mummy needs some sleep,' mumbled Power, who had snatched just two hours and 17 minutes of shuteye since setting off from Malin Head at the northerly tip of Ireland.

In the days succeeding her record attempt Power was once more flooded with messages from women. They were inspired by the symbol of not only a woman but also a mother, achieving an incredible feat of endurance just three years after the birth of her third child. A mother who trained by walking 12,000 steps during the daily school run and a mother who refused to feel guilty during her Ireland recovery when the kids spent a few too many hours watching television while she ate chocolate cake and napped. Power demonstrated that with the right support, women were far more than caregivers, they were made to last. With sex-appropriate training and the same opportunity to participate as men, imagine what more women could do.

19.
TRAIN LIKE A GIRL

As she prepared to walk out to the starting point, Vriko Kwok felt a familiar dampness in her underwear. Only minutes earlier she had slipped into her tight brown shorts, confident the bespoke racing kit would support her six-day challenge. Standing under the searing Californian sun, the sticky feeling between her legs threatened to change everything. All the 4am training runs in Hong Kong could be for nothing. Having her period arrive early was not part of the plan.

Kwok had been under the scrutiny of running coaches, sports scientists, nutritionists and psychologists for the past 12 months, yet this had taken her by surprise. She was about to embark on the biggest physical and mental challenge of her life, and now she had something else to deal with. A year ago, the 30-year-old had never run, scared off at a young age by the school bullies who laughed at her size. 'I hated running because I never saw myself doing it. I got bullied quite badly growing up and that put me off running for a long time.' Now, she was about to run alongside nine of the world's best ultra-marathon runners in an attempt to go from zero to 300km. Everything was riding on this moment. Her training, her self-belief, her determination to prove the cynics wrong. She must not waiver. Menstrual cycle or not, this Hong Kong entrepreneur was not going to quit before she started. Deciding it was a natural part of being a woman, Kwok declined to take a pill to stop her period and leaned into the experience. It was not like she was alone. Three of the other female athletes began menstruating during the 2024 Lululemon Further event, which sought to measure the impact of endurance on women's bodies.

Collectively, the global team of women ran 4,636km across the six days, with a US ultra runner, Camille Herron, setting 13 records, while she covered 901km on the 4.12km loop. The first-of-its-kind research project sought to break new horizons for women in ultra sport (see more in Chapter 20) through race gear innovation and data collection. This had been sorely lacking in sports science owing to the patriarchal structure in research and innovation (see Chapter 8). The Further initiative hoped to begin solving the puzzle of how women could be supported to endure – and where their limits lay. As the novice of the pack Kwok, a former Brazilian Jiu-jitsu player, became the symbol of possibility, proving what a woman could achieve with the right training and support. With a heavy build habituated to martial arts combat, Kwok required a massive shift in lifestyle to adapt her body to long-distance running. For a year she worked with the Canadian Sport Institute Pacific, training, eating and sleeping like an ultra runner. Externally, she was kitted out with personalised clothing, designed to meet her specific ergonomic requirements. Internally, her body's energy needs were calculated by a team of sports scientists. Early tests identified she had severe anaemia, meaning she was able to quickly address the iron deficiency and boost her energy levels. She worked closely with a coach who created an individualised training schedule to fit around her busy working life. A nutritionist helped her to lose nine kilograms of weight while stressing the importance of maximising calorie intake during long runs. Armed with the correct preparation and knowledge for her body type and sex, Kwok began the Further event with the belief and assurance that she could complete an ultra marathon a day, for six consecutive days, no matter her background. She had just as much right to be there as her record-breaking teammates. They were all pushing progress forward, testing the limits and redefining female possibility. It was the perfect demonstration of what women could achieve with the same level of funding and infrastructure as men. But the Lululemon Further campaign also highlighted a juxtaposition within sport.

While the 10 athletes had the finest minds in sport science to support their training, six-day run, and recovery, the event was also a mass data-gathering exercise. On the one hand, the message conveyed that women could achieve remarkable feats when trained within an appropriate framework. Conversely, it highlighted that scientists lack sufficient knowledge about women's bodies in terms of training for, participating in, and recovering from ultra-endurance sports. Therein lies the paradox.

If the scientific and coaching community recognise that women have different training requirements than men, but most research has been conducted on young, white males, how can women be best informed when it comes to training? And how can we really know if they are capable of becoming faster than men, the longer the distance? Take sports injury risk, for example. A wealth of studies have established that women are disproportionately impacted by knee and hip osteoarthritis which increases the risk of traumatic knee injury, particularly to the anterior cruciate ligament, which is common amongst footballers. But research has failed to examine how sex factors might explain this disparity, and rehabilitation programmes do not address the physical and psychological factors that might contribute to women's worse outcomes. When women athletes return to competition after giving birth to a child there is little evidence to guide them. This can result in decreased performance and increased risk of injury despite positive cardiovascular adaptations (Chapter 12). The sport science community does not know nearly enough about how to train female athletes.

Stacy Sims, a female exercise physiologist, has made it her life's work to help women train according to their physiology. As a triathlete and nutrition scientist, she has pushed back against the status quo of research which focuses on men. Driven by 'unfairness and injustice' in sport science, she strives to develop training targeted to women. 'When I started down this path, I realised that all the training and nutritional recommendations had been generalised,' Sims says. 'Yet we know there are sex differences from birth with muscle morphology, women's endurance, and metabolism. In ultra endurance, women are meeting the men. They're catching up or surpassing men and it's not the biomechanical aspect. It's the fact that women are more enduring, both mentally and physically. But when I went into the research it was all so patriarchal.' Sims argues that women need to train differently to men for endurance, by dropping training volume and increasing intensity. The women who come to her clinic are often overtrained, immune deficient and have low energy availability. Her approach favours lactate threshold work, explosive plyometric workouts and strength training rather than the traditional approach of 80 per cent of training performed at low intensity and 20 per cent at high intensity.

Women also need a different approach to sport-specific fuelling, Sims says. Following the recommended guidance of carbohydrates per hour does not necessarily translate across the sexes. Women tend to use a greater relative proportion of fats during endurance exercise and their metabolic rate changes throughout the month based on ovulation, and regardless of physical activity. The minimum requirements for female ultra-endurance athletes, particularly those who are small and lean, are much higher. Then there is the problem of 'shrink it and pink it' sports nutrition. Relying on sports gels and products containing fructose and maltodextrin is a big mistake, says Sims, because they overload the intestines, leading to gastrointestinal stress which women are far more prone to. The post-activity recovery window is also much smaller for women. To maximise muscle adaption, they need to eat protein within 45 minutes of finishing, while men can afford to wait longer. Sims vehemently asserts that all areas of training need to be viewed via a female lens from recovery periods to sleep cycles to hydration techniques, and beyond.

Yet the science, product development and coaching are decades behind practice, making it difficult for athletes to understand what the best approach is. There simply aren't any tried and tested guidelines for women, making coaches afraid to deviate from the established norm. There isn't even agreement amongst female sports scientists. 'There's a lot of voices in this space now but there is definitely some questionable stuff out there,' says a leading UK sports dietician, Renee McGregor, author of More Fuel You. 'I think what they're [some other researchers] intending on doing is amazing in that they're trying to raise awareness of women, and help to make change, but in terms of scientific knowledge, I would question some of it,' she says. 'Some people in this space are very specific about what women should do. In terms of saying on day seven you must eat x amount of protein and x amount of carbohydrate, then 100 per cent no, we can't be saying that. And if anybody is telling you that, they're wrong. We just don't have the science behind that.'

So many variables make it hard to unpack what is having an impact on the nervous system, and in turn performance. 'I think most scientists are underestimating the impact of threat and stress on our nervous system,' says McGregor. 'It's quite a difficult thing to measure. Our body picks up on threat, but you're not always going to necessarily understand if that's a threat due to dehydration, poor sleep, not fuelling properly or not getting enough of a certain type of nutrient. It's a complicated picture.' At least with male athletes there is a baseline of data to extrapolate from, but the same cannot be said for females. McGregor explains: 'When you're working with a male athlete you can start by saying the majority of studies suggest this is going to happen. So, from a nutrition point we'll start with x amount of carbs and protein. There's no one size fits all and it's hugely individualised but at least for men there's always ballpark figures we can work with. But in females, we don't even have that, we're always using data from studies on white, trained, young men.'

While Sims and McGregor may take a different approach to working with female athletes, they both agree that the biggest issue in women's training is the mismatch between calories eaten and calories burned during exercise. This condition known as Relative Energy Deficiency in Sport (REDs) is common in both sexes but far more prevalent in women, particularly at the elite level. Evidence suggests most males can sustain a lower energy availability for longer than females before physiological and psychological disturbances manifest.

Ultra-endurance athletes are at relatively high risk of REDs because they often train for more than 30 hours per week, burning through tens of thousands of calories. Alarmingly, a survey of more than 300 ultra runners found that half of athletes restricted calories – which can be partially attributed to the rising popularity of low carbohydrate, high fat or high protein diets. For women, this can have serious health consequences with amenorrhea (menstrual dysfunction) being one of the most common symptoms. Female athletes with low energy availability can have disrupted menstrual cycles, or stop having periods altogether, a sign that the body is energy depleted. Menstrual dysfunction may also be related to stress fractures which disproportionately affect women. Despite this, many women have normalised losing their period, with up to 40 per cent of female athletes experiencing menstrual cycle disorders. 'I think the biggest problem is we know that most women under-consume because of fear of putting weight on or having the right body composition. We've always assumed that the optimal body composition for women is that lower is better. We've pushed women into these teeny, tiny body compositions, which then means they are not menstruating, they're not healthy, and lo and behold, they can't maintain their performances for more than a year or two,' says McGregor. One of the indicators of low energy availability is a low iron count, something which is naturally more prevalent in women due to blood loss during menstruation. To prevent iron deficiency, female athletes may require around 10mg more a day than the recommended (patriarchal) dose of 14mg, according to a recent study.

Rather than being a weakness, having a regular period is a good indicator that the body is getting enough nutrients to support training, is adapting to physical stress and is well rested. Just how sensitive the body is to hormonal changes is both widely variable, and understudied, making guidance for training a complex matter. McGregor says: 'While we know that hormonal changes do influence our nutritional intake it is still so individualised because our menstrual cycle is so affected by lifestyle factors. No one's really doing the science. Personally, I don't think we know enough about the menstrual cycle or hormones.'

Tracking the menstrual cycle has become the latest fitness trend with women syncing their workouts to their menstruation phase. A quick glance at a hormone app can indicate whether it's a good day to focus on a fast run, hit the weights in the gym or to conserve energy at a yoga class. Cycle syncing promises to boost optimal fitness and reduce injury risk by aligning workouts with the follicular and luteal phases of menstruation and ovulation. And while hormone levels do fluctuate during the menstruation cycle causing shifts in energy levels, mood and stress, how this impacts women's power and endurance is currently unquantifiable. Factors such as sleep, stress, food and motivation could have a bigger impact on performance than the phase of the menstrual cycle. Then there are the women on contraceptive medication which stops their periods, meaning they are unable to track their cycles. Every woman is different. There is no phase of the menstrual cycle when it is harmful to exercise, and some women thrive at the start of their period, while others feel at their weakest. There is merit in monitoring symptoms at different phases of the cycle, and adapting workouts according to how an athlete feels, but coaches need to tailor a plan to an individual rather than follow a one-size-fits-all approach, says McGregor. As Kwok and her three Further teammates demonstrated, hormones can be unpredictable, but they don't have to dictate performance.

It would be naïve, however, to suggest that menstruating through an endurance race has no impact on the body. Kwok had to make adjustments. She was fortunate enough to have the help of a large contingent of experts who were monitoring all manner of metrics including her core (basal) body temperature. At the start of each day, Kwok would swallow a core temperature pill which gradually passed through her system. Armed with the right knowledge she could make subtle changes to her hydration, nutrition and kit, which enabled her to keep running day after day.

As luck would have it, starting her period was perhaps a blessing in disguise. While women's basal body temperature rises in the second half of the menstruation cycle during and after ovulation (luteal phase), when progesterone levels drop during menstruation, the basal temperature typically falls, returning to the baseline level seen during the follicular phase. Having a raised core body temperature makes it easier to become dehydrated but can also make women more susceptible to sodium loss. A rise in progesterone levels in the days leading up to a period can have an impact on kidney function and the regulation of electrolytes including sodium. This can also cause fluid retention and increased plasma volume, diluting the amount of sodium in the blood. All these changes in the body make it easier to lose sodium through sweat when exercising, potentially putting women at increased risk of hyponatremia (low sodium levels) during this phase of their cycle. Add to the mix running in hot conditions and it becomes clear that women need to pay extra attention to their hydration and electrolyte balance when exercising.

In general, women's core body temperature rises more quickly than men's during exercise but they sweat less and have relatively less body fluid. Since hydration has a cooling effect on the body, drinking enough fluid is arguably more important for female endurance athletes. For Kwok, this was a difficult task given that the Further course sat in a barren landscape devoid of shade where ground temperatures rose to 30 degrees Celsius in the mid-afternoon sun. With the Santa Rosa mountains looming on one side and the shady palm tree groves tantalisingly out of reach on the other, the runners had the thankless task of moving under the full heat of the sun. To add insult to injury, Kwok had to run continuous laps past the invitingly fresh waters of Lake Lahuilla for six days. To avoid the worst of the heat, Kwok rose at 4am each morning to start running before napping in the afternoon. She then began running again in the early evening until 10pm, with the aim of completing 50km per day. This strategy, together with a targeted hydration regime, helped her body to thermoregulate despite the internal and external heat challenges.

Another aid in her toolkit was the first-of-its-kind cooling system designed specifically for women by Lululemon. During their research and development the company worked with female athletes to understand their body temperature needs. Women were asking for a garment which helped them to manage their body temperature, and correctly and comfortably fitted their bust. Lululemon created an ice vest which fitted like a running pack but could be loaded up with ice in targeted cooling zones at the front and back. The insulated pouches slowed the ice from melting meaning the women could run for longer before having to stop to replenish. The close fit also held the ice right next to the body. Together with UV cooling ice sleeves, ice neck bandana and cooling headwear, these became an essential piece of kit for the Further runners.

Regulating temperature during endurance feats is of particular importance to women because they can be more significantly impacted by heat strain than men. But that's only half the story. With the right training and acclimation heat does not have to be an obstacle for women. Puck Alkemade, an environmental exercise physiologist, spent her PhD thesis studying the influence of heat strain in exercise performance and the strategies that can help the body acclimate. While at the University of Amsterdam she studied responses in different athlete groups including recreational athletes, Olympic and Paralympic athletes and athletes with a spinal cord injury. She is acutely aware that most physiology research is performed with male participants and her study went some way towards redressing the balance. What she discovered was fascinating. While women and men can both successfully adapt to heat stress, they do so in a different way. Alkemade said: 'We found that smaller individuals with low body mass who were typically females, had a large heart rate adaption, whereas larger individuals with a high body mass, who were typically male, had a large sweat adaptation. So, both groups adapted albeit in different ways and it didn't result in any differences in their performance improvement.' Alkemade also argues that it is not being female or male that impacts thermoregulation (the biological mechanism that maintains a steady internal body temperature) but rather body dimensions. Larger people are typically men and sweating is their body's preferred way to lose heat, while smaller people who are typically women, experience heat loss via the widening of blood vessels in the skin (vasodilation). This becomes an advantage for smaller, typically female, athletes during hot and humid conditions where sweat cannot evaporate due to the moisture in the air, and vasodilation is far more effective. In hot and dry conditions skin heat loss is less beneficial, putting most women at a disadvantage.

This is where technology has a role to play. Wearing a cooling device to lower skin temperature such as sleeves enables hotter heat from the body's core to move more easily and escape, which in turn decreases heat strain. While research into the impact of heat during different phases of the menstrual cycle is largely inconclusive, female athletes can take a personalised approach to measuring core body temperature. This no longer relies on taking the type of pill ingested by Kwok, which was originally designed for male astronauts. Tech is now reaching the mass market enabling athletes and coaches to collate female-centric data. Leading the charge is CORE, a wearable app which can monitor basal body temperature fluctuations throughout the menstrual cycle, enabling female athletes to assess whether exercise performance or training readiness is influenced by rising and falling core body temperature.

Companies like CORE are incorporating sex difference research, and hiring physiologists like Alkemade, to better understand the training requirements of female athletes. But they are still very much the outliers in a multi-billion global industry obsessed with male performance. Product innovation leans heavily towards male morphology with sports shoe design being one of the biggest culprits. Worth approximately $133 billion, the sports shoe industry is happy to keep churning out standardised shoes based on the shape of men's feet. Breaking the mould is Brit Martin Dean, a sportswear disruptor, who has developed the lace-less QLVR sports shoe with manufacturing processes based on the specific biomechanics of women. 'The majority of all athletic footwear is made to fit a man's foot shape, then downscaled to women's sizes on that same tooling to save on production costs,' explains Dean who has spent 30 years designing footwear. 'The use of the lace allows this to work to a degree because the laces can take up the slack. But women's feet are anatomically shaped differently to men's; they are narrower at the heel, have a higher instep and a wider toe box, so the majority of women's training shoes are just small men's shoes.'

The reluctance of brands to overhaul their tooling to create female and male apparatus is because it would bring into question the products they already have on the market, he claims. As a start-up company, Dean didn't have this marketing dilemma and he could focus on his dream of creating a lace-less shoe, overcoming anatomical differences along the way. 'I think I've been obsessed with hands-free trainers since seeing the boots in the film Back To The Future as a kid. I was baffled by the fact that despite the amount of innovation in sports footwear in the past 50 years, designers were still relying on a piece of string to fasten them.' When developing the QLVR prototype Dean realised his bespoke fit system would not suit a woman's foot.

'The current unisex fit system means it would have been too loose on the back of a woman's foot. That's when we realised that the majority of footwear is made to fit a man's foot. So we decided to launch it for women. That's not to say we wouldn't offer it to men down the line, but it would be using different tooling.' While his intentions appear to be making progress for women it hasn't stopped critics from claiming the QLVR shoe is patronising. 'People were being brutal about it online claiming we designed a shoe without laces for women because we think women can't tie their shoelaces.'

While unjustified, the ridicule Dean faced points to a deep-seated problem within sport. Women's endurance sport is dominated by male coaches who often base their advice and training techniques on what has gone before. The status quo continues as coaches rely on methods designed for men, underpinned by research primarily conducted on men. When presented with the opportunity to upskill their knowledge around female athletes, male coaches can be reticent. When researchers at the La Trobe University in Australia invited coaches working with female athletes to complete a short online course on considerations for female athletes, they received far greater uptake from women. Out of the whole cohort, 72 per cent were female and just 28 per cent men. It was expected that more men might participate in the course since globally there are significantly more males than females working as women's sports coaches. The researchers concluded that women in coaching were more aware of their lack of knowledge and actively sought out this information, while male coaches adopted a one-size-fits-all coaching practice that was not adapted to sex differences. But in order to truly individualise and optimise training these differences must be considered by coaches, say Kirsty Elliott-Sale and Guy Pitchers in a seminal paper, Considerations for Coaches Training Female Athletes. The paper urges coaches to understand female-specific issues such as the menstrual cycle, breast health, female psychology and trends in female injuries so that women can be trained in their own right and not grouped in with men.

Coaches do indeed need to understand these female-specific issues. How women respond to training and competition is underpinned by sex differences in goal orientation and sources of confidence, plus additional stressors of gender stereotypes, unequal treatment and patronising attitudes. Female athletes are far more likely to experience sexual harassment, heightening their anxiety and negatively impacting their self-esteem. Women in sport are treated differently by society, whether it's Kwok's experience of being told she was 'too fat to run', or Sims' realisation of the gender inequity of sport science research. Sportswomen need to be coached and trained in their own right and not grouped with men. As participation gradually increases in female endurance events, sports medicine clinicians need to understand the medical conditions affecting them.

...

Women also need safe spaces to train in, and a community which bolsters their confidence. For Kwok, this community came from her peers, who were able to offer her guidance based on their own lived-in experience, rather than garnered from endurance textbooks with a male bias. Her teammates stressed the importance of learning how to eat on the move and gave advice on how to consume up to 4,000 calories a day. 'Every morning without fail, I had avocado with poached eggs and two slices of bacon – which I hadn't eaten for 25 years. But one of my teammates said the sodium and fat were really good for ultra running,' says Kwok. The Further ten also gave each other moral support and companionship during the six-day event, teaming up with one another for at least one lap to stave off the feeling of isolation.

This sense of community and achieving a shared goal is the key to female success according to an ultra-running endurance coach, Hannah Walsh. Each year she coaches a group of 10 women in her Breaking 250 initiative. The British mentor takes women with little running experience through a programme of training to complete their first multi-day 250k ultra overseas. She creates a safe space where women can be vulnerable, ask questions and share what they are juggling in their daily lives. 'In my experience, the best way to get women into the sport is to give them the support that they need to do it, through that small close knit group community. Most of the women say they never would have attempted anything like this without the support of the group and they never would have believed that they could do something like this without the support of the group. We can spend two hours on a call during the programme talking about managing hygiene while on your period during long-distance races,' says Walsh. Many of her clients are menopausal, a prolonged period when women's bodies are in an immense state of flux.

Walsh's athletes share strategies for coping with physiological changes brought on by the decline of oestrogen levels. Menopause can significantly impact female endurance athletes in various ways affecting their performance, recovery and overall health. Bone density decreases, along with muscle mass and strength. Hormonal changes can lead to changes in metabolism and a reduction of cardiovascular performance. The body's ability to regulate temperature is impacted leading to increased heat intolerance. Sleep, which is crucial for recovery, can be disturbed. Training adjustments are required to mitigate the impact of all these changes, with a greater focus on strength training, interval sessions, increased protein intake and sleep management. While the research literature adequately understands the effect of menopause on athletic performance, most sporting bodies do not provide coaching guidance on practical support for female Masters athletes (aged over 35).

Whether it is women's approach to nutrition, training or kit, the best approach we currently have relies heavily on trial and error. The science is slowly seeping through, but the data is limited. As a result, the guidelines and coaching techniques have been slow to adapt and there is still so much to learn.

20.
UNSTOPPABLE

The child spots a flash of red through the trees and runs up the rough road, excitedly yelling 'she's here'. Murmurs ripple through the small spread-out crowd lining the forest track. They crane their necks to see if the youngster is right, the atmosphere tense. They are either about to witness history or crushing disappointment. Is she coming, can she do it? There are only two minutes left on the clock now. Then all of a sudden, the onlookers begin whooping and clapping. Jasmin Paris is running up the tarmac as fast as she possibly can for someone at the end of a 100-mile-plus battle in the mountains. She is using her whole body to propel herself forward. This petite 40-year-old woman, running poles loose in her hands, is breathing hard, head bobbing, her skin almost grey. Clearly at her absolute limits, she storms up the final bit of gradient. Paris does not appear to notice the bystanders now cheering her on with all their might. Her steely focus is on finishing. Every single person is willing her onwards, sure they are watching one of the greatest achievements ever seen in ultra endurance. She collapses over the large pale yellow gate that signals the end of her race, before dropping to the ground gasping deeply for oxygen. Seemingly on the verge of passing out, she slumps against a wall before moving to lie on her side with her eyes shut.

Paris attempts to recover as her husband watches over anxiously and cameras flash. In March 2024, with just 90 seconds to spare, Paris becomes the first woman ever to complete the Barkley Marathons in its 38-year history. It is a race so notoriously tough that its founder, a colourful character called Gary 'Lazarus Lake' Cantrell, once said no woman would be able to complete it. He later qualified his view to say if any woman could finish the Barkley, it would be Paris. The ultra-endurance legend from Edinburgh, who loves nothing more than to run around in the mountains, has once again stunned the ultra-running world and beyond, by doing the seemingly impossible. This book opened with Paris breaking the Winter Spine record, running up the mountainous Pennine way from the Peak District in England to its conclusion in Scotland. When looking for what would come next, it is no surprise she set her sights on Tennessee for one of the most unique and devilish events ever devised.

...

For the 40 runners who get to compete in the annual Barkley Marathons in Frozen Head State Park by personal invitation, there is no GPS or tracking device to guide them through the tricky terrain. They only have a basic compass and their own notes taken from the rough map they were allowed to see before the start. Cantrell or 'Laz' as he is affectionately known and a friend, Karl 'Raw Dog' Henn, came up with the concept after hearing about the tale of an escaped convict. Locked up in nearby Bushy State Penitentiary after killing Martin Luther King Jr, James Earl Ray broke out and ran around the woods for 55 hours trying to hide. When he was finally caught, he had only moved about 12 miles. Hearing the story, Cantrell calculated he could have run 100 miles and the idea was born. Since the first version in 1986, the route has changed every year with Cantrell delighting in making it harder. So that runners know the time, he hands out cheap watches with quirks that make them difficult to read. The race can start at any point of Cantrell's choosing, which he does by lighting a cigarette, at which point competitors have 60 hours to do five 20-ish mile loops. To prove they have done the full route (which is largely inaccessible to any support crew even if they were allowed one, which they're not), they must tear out specific pages of books hidden along the course. The direction of each loop also changes between clockwise and anticlockwise as the runners progress.

The terrain is unforgiving. Barkley marathoners must tackle more than 16,000 metres of vertical climb with very few paths. Along the way there are various hidden rocky cliffs and waist-high brambles that carve deep scratches on their limbs. Obstacles to overcome include Danger Dave's climbing wall and Rat Jaw; a steep slope covered in razor-sharp saw briars that slash through clothing. Up until 2018, more than half of races had ended without a single runner finishing. Since 1989, when the full 100-mile version was in place, only 20 of the 1,000 runners who have attempted it have made it to the end, albeit a handful more than once. Cantrell's goal is to make sure the Barkley is 'at the very horizon of human potential'. To be one of the few invited to enter you have to write an essay on 'Why I should be allowed to run the Barkley'. If selected, it seems fitting that the runner receives a 'letter of condolence'.

Barely any women had come close to Paris's achievement in the almost four decades of Barkley history. Before Paris did it in 2022, only four women had ever completed the 'fun run' of three loops. Paris had come the furthest in 2023 when she started loop four but did not meet the cut-off to start the final section. One other female runner, Sue Johnston, had also started the fourth loop in 2001 but got no further. After the 2024 race, when the photographs had been taken of the five competitors who managed to finish, Paris admitted she had been on the verge of passing out. She would either reach that gate or collapse on the ground in front of it trying. Her blurry vision had blocked out her surroundings, the roar of the crowd creating a tunnel of noise. For Paris, running 100 miles at any other point would be a walk in the park. Yet here the terrain literally stops runners in their tracks. Paris described slopes so steep you slide back down them and places where competitors are essentially climbing on their bellies. The only sleep she had was a quick power nap before the final loop. This time, in addition to the usual animals that her sleep-deprived brain vividly hallucinated, she saw sinister figures in black Mackintoshes.

Fuelling herself with as much regular food as she could, including rice pudding, sandwiches, porridge and bananas, she also had nasty gut problems to contend with. By the end she was struggling to eat at all. Her mantra in those final hours, when she desperately wanted to stop, was to tell herself she did not want to come and do it again. 'I still find it really exciting to push myself, especially when I don't know whether I can do something. It sounds a bit corny, but you also find out more about yourself, when you strip away all the stuff that makes life easier,' she said afterwards.

A founding member of the Green Runners and with two young children, Paris is mindful of her time and carbon footprint. When she signs up to an event, it will be one that really counts. She has to be 'all in'. The attraction of the Barkley was solely that the race was seen as undoable. After her first try in 2022, she thought to herself: 'This is possible, it's just going to take a lot of work'. So, she put in the work, as she had done previously for the Montane Winter Spine Race (see Chapter 1).

Paris trained from 5am to 7am every morning and completed multiple strength sessions a week to shore up her dodgy left knee that had no anterior cruciate ligament. Once on the course, her experience meant this time she was able to pre-empt problems or correct them before they were race-ending. However all that training and preparation did not stop 'every fibre of her being' screaming at her to stop running as she ploughed to that finish line with less than two minutes to spare. 'I've never had to dig so deep.' Paris, who received an MBE (an award from the British crown in recognition of outstanding achievement) for her efforts, has no intention of doing the Barkley again because she has proven she can. It is time to move on. Next stop is the Tor des Geants in the Italian Alps.

...

Throughout the process of writing this book, women all over the world have continuously broken barriers and records, won races and set themselves new ultra challenges. At the time of writing, Lael Wilcox (Chapter 10) has just broken the female solo Round the World cycling record where riders must cover a minimum of 29,000 km (18,000 miles). A key detail to her adventure – which fans followed closely on social media over 108 days, 12 hours, and 12 minutes – is that she chose a more challenging route than she could have done because she loves riding in the mountains so much. She was not driven by ego or a desire to be the best, because this would have dictated a faster, easier route. It was about the journey.

In April 2024, Sarah Perry spent the Easter holidays smashing the women's record on the South West Coast Path as well as achieving the fastest overall self-supported time. Running 630 miles from Dorset to Somerset on the longest national trail in England in 13 days 11 hours and 31 minutes, she knocked two hours off the previous record set by David Myers. She has cited her 'meticulous planning' as being key to the endeavour. An awe-inspiring athlete, Perry battled the elements, covered the equivalent of four Mount Everests, trudged through the worst mud she had ever seen and did plenty of all-nighters. Her advice for others looking to take on challenges was 'dream big and don't forget the spreadsheet.'

Her success had come just weeks after setting a new British record for the longest Backyard Ultra by a woman, running 170 miles over 41 laps. Perry has described the format, in which each four-mile loop has to be completed in an hour, as 'fascinating' because in her experience the usual gender stereotypes do not apply. 'As long as you've got endurance and can manage sleep deprivation, you have a shot at going far in a Backyard Ultra.' In October the same year, she proved this again by completing 59 laps, totalling 245.8 miles, over two and a half days, beating her own record. She was the last runner standing. After the event, the organisers put a post on social media stating: 'Anyone can win a backyard ultra'. While their intentions were to celebrate the outcome of the event, many felt that the post diminished Perry's achievement and women's success in endurance. Language matters and it shows there is still much work to do.

Taming the winter storms, a Utah-based adventurer, Sunny Stroeer, became the first woman to complete the Iditarod Trail Invitational in Alaska on skis. The world's longest winter ultra-marathon, it takes up to a month to complete. Stroeer joined four men to be the first group to ever do the 1,000-mile route solely on skis. People might usually opt for a fat bike, which has extra wide tyres for traversing snow, or even do the route by dog sled. It took German-born Stroeer 29 days, 21 hours and 55 minutes to complete the trail, which involved trekking through the iciest of conditions dragging her kit behind her. Temperatures can drop to -45 degrees Celsius and for a 200-mile stretch in the Alaskan wilderness she did not see anyone else at all. Conditions are so brutal that if something goes wrong, rescue may not be possible.

On the sea, at the very start of the year, a team of four ultra athletes from Nottingham completed a record-breaking row across the Atlantic. In 2024, they became the fastest British women to row from La Gomera to Antigua, doing it in under 40 days. They rowed for 14 hours a day, sometimes through thunder and lightning storms, to inspire more girls and women to take part. Over the two years of training, the 'There She Rows' team campaigned and raised money for gender equality in sport. In the same race – called the World's Toughest Row – a team of women from Jersey became the oldest female crew to row any ocean. Aged between 55 and 60 years, they broke the world record with a time of 58 days 12 hours and 30 minutes at sea.

Other record attempts have not gone as hoped. Ellen Falterman, who also goes by the name Ellen Magellan, has been attempting to be the first person to circumnavigate the globe purely by rowing. The Texan had to abandon attempts in 2022 and 2024 because of family bearevements and damage to her boat. She intends to keep trying.

To crown a phenomenal year of ultra achievement, the US ultra runner Tara Dower took 13 hours and 32 minutes off the Appalachian trail record in 2024 to achieve the fastest known time – for a woman or man. She averaged 54 miles a day over 40 days to cover the 2197.4 miles of mountain range that runs from Maine to Georgia. Along the way she raised $20,000 for Girls on the Run, a charity that encourages young girls to gain confidence and 'find the joy' in running. 'My hope is to inspire women and girls to go for that tough goal no matter if it's with running or in life,' she said on reaching the finish.

In the long and far from exhaustive list above, some have beaten men's records, some women's records. Some have done a feat no one else has ever even attempted. They are all fulfilling their potential. Pushing their limits, learning as they go and trying again. It does seem that increasing numbers of women are excelling in ultra-endurance sport. But it is not just an artefact of journalists realising that headlines celebrating female success get a lot of attention. There is data to back it up. Ultra marathon statistics held by the most comprehensive database, the DUV, show that women from China, Brazil, the USA, Hong Kong, Sweden, France, the UK, Spain and more won races outright in 2024. Last person standing races, Backyard Ultras, non-stop trail races, six to 24-hour events, 30, 50, 100 and 200-milers around the world have all recorded female winners ahead of men. The official list has more than 400 recorded for the first nine months of the year. Every year the figure ticks upwards. And the detailed global database tracks back decades.

In 1980, when Edwards, Trason, Robinson and Dodds (see Chapter 4) were finding their feet in this little-known sport, four ultra races had been won outright by a female athlete. As the sport has grown in popularity, the number of races has also expanded as has the proportion of women competing. By 2000, 16 women had won an event outright across the USA, Canada, Australia, Italy, Germany and Austria. A decade later the figure was 103 and by 2023 there were 660. The database, which covers official races, not fastest known times or world records, lists 2,000 female outright winners since its records began.

...

As more women reach the start line and see others achieving, these accomplishments will grow further. It is an exciting time for female ultra-endurance sport. After the success of the all-female She Ultra race in North Wales in 2024 (see Chapter 18), 700 women registered for the following year's event. It clearly demonstrates that when women are provided with appropriate support they become unstoppable. And as they continue to push beyond what they thought was possible for themselves, a growing team of coaches, physiotherapists, race directors, support crew and scientists are learning more about how they can achieve their best.

When the sportswear brand Lululemon announced its Further initiative to run a six-day women's ultra marathon, it was not just about breaking records (see Chapter 19). It set out to see what could happen if the women taking part had access to all the support, resources and product innovation that male athletes get as a matter of course. In addition to demonstrating how far women could go when provided with the right conditions to achieve their best results, it also sought to explore the scientific evidence regarding whether women excel in endurance activities. It wanted to answer those key questions around whether women have more fatigue resistance (Chapter 10) and find the limit of female energy expenditure (Chapter 11).

Ten women ran round a certified looped course at Lake Cahuilla in La Quinta, California, to set personal, world distance and time records. To meet the challenge, Lululemon came up with 36 new kit innovations backed by research in collaboration with the athletes. This included the Beyondfeel Women's Running Shoe, which the company said had been designed around the shape of a female foot, as well as clothing that was comfortable with storage for fuel and water.

Chantelle Murnaghan, vice president of research and product innovation, explains that when the team was developing the idea for the Further initiative it realised there was a dearth of evidence to inform its work. The team was spurred on to push the boundaries and 'really start to question' the understanding of female sports science. It took on a life of its own because of the passion of those in the team and outside researchers who 'jumped on board' to bring their expertise in particular areas. 'They all wanted to push this understanding as well,' Murnaghan says. Not only did they identify ways to better support the female runners doing the event over the six days, through kit design and tailored nutrition, they also took constant measurements and feedback during the event. It ended up being 'one of the most comprehensive in-race data collections that has ever been done to my knowledge,' according to Murnaghan. Unlike a research project in academia where researchers are focused on a very specific narrow topic, they were able to explore everything from biomechanics to energy expenditure to psychosocial aspects.

Some of the most vital bits of kit the team developed were around keeping the women runners cool as they did laps of the dusty track in the intense dry heat. When it forecasted what the main barriers to success in the run would be, thermal regulation was a big one. Over the course of the six-day event, temperatures were expected to swing from 30 degrees Celsius in the middle of the day down to quite cool in the evening. The women would also need to be protected from the elements if it started to rain. It turned out to be very useful planning as every single one of these extremes happened on day one. Meanwhile, a nutritionist documented everything the runners consumed and monitored their energy intake and usage. The team also measured the biomechanics of the female runners through the shoes and force plates embedded in the track itself. Foot scans were done and urine and blood samples collected, in addition to cognitive tests on the runners' mental state. Neuromuscular fatigue testing checked how their legs were holding up. Records were kept of menstrual cycles in the run-up to and during the event.

Collectively, the ten runners completed more than 2,880 miles. Camille Herron was the headline grabber. The tenacious 43-year-old US ultra runner has always taken a scientific approach to her running. Describing herself as a 'data geek,' she has a spreadsheet that calculates how far she has run since she began in 1995. At the time of writing, she is at 111,381.75 lifetime running miles.

Diagnosed the year before with autism and ADHD, a lot of things that make her an excellent ultra runner, have now started to make more sense, including her tendency to be hyper-focused. When the Further project was announced, Herron remarked the further she goes, the stronger she is. 'This is a sport where women can excel,' she said. 'We're winning races outright. We're breaking men's records. More women need to know that. We are made to endure.' She was speaking just a month after breaking the men's course record at a trail marathon in Texas. She is the first athlete to have won all three road IAU World Championships for 50K, 100K and 24 hours. Among a long list of firsts, she was the first ultra runner to win both the Comrades Marathon and Spartathlon and in 2023, she became the first woman to break 24 hours at the latter.

At the Further event, with the support and research teams meeting her every need, Herron toppled record after record, adding 12 more to her collection. Over the six days, she ran 560.29 miles (901.71km), beating the women's world best of 549 miles that had been set in

1990. Her remarkable tally included the 300, 400 and 500-mile world records and the three, four, and five-day records.

Support from a sports psychologist helped her learn more about how her neurodivergence enables her to push through pain, fatigue and sleep deprivation. Other than some swelling, her legs held up well, she said. Not shy about sharing what this level of endurance does to the body, she had her period to contend with from day two as well as losing control of her bladder and bowels. Her gut held up well with regular food and she only vomited once on the first day.

Herron has described the level of support she had from the specialists at the event as 'magical'. They calculated exactly what she needed to get to the next record. Herron crossed the finish line to Madonna's Vogue and still had the energy to start dancing. While she is excited to see the science that will come out, she also wants to find out how far she can go without it being an experiment. 'I think I can break the men's world record,' she said. 'I think that we know enough people in the world now that we can work on optimising all the variables and create the optimal situation to go for the men's record.'

A cynic could view the Lululemon project as a marketing exercise. Certainly, some on social media criticised its lavishness and elaborate publicity. But it was never about doing research for the company's own purposes, says Murnaghan. A key output was to encourage others to follow along with additional questions and additional investigations. 'It is not just about getting the answers from this particular event and after the event but being a spark to kind of push others to explore research in their own areas and beyond.' Records are of course made to be broken and a few months on from Further, Danish female ultra athlete Stine Rex notched up another seven miles on top of Herron's six-day record. Female endurance athletes continue to progress, pushing ever onward.

...

The research is also pushing forwards. For the first time ever, Team USA elite female athletes have been asked their opinion on research. Extraordinarily, until now their voices have not been heard even when determining research agendas to elevate female athletic performance and wellbeing. The survey of female sports stars identified 14 topics for future research, with the top five being menstrual cycle symptoms, recovery, birth control, mental health, and fuelling and the menstrual cycle. Tellingly, institutionalised sexism was also identified as an area that required further investigation. These results will now lay the foundation for future sports science research to begin to address the gap in gender parity.

In the world of ultra endurance, two of the researchers highlighted in this book, Camilla Illidi (Chapter 8) and Nick Tiller (Chapters 7 and 11), have recently published a paper on sex differences in two ultra marathons that had comparable numbers of male and female competitors. In a 50-mile event of 96 finishers, they found no difference in median time overall between the sexes, but the top ten men finished faster than the top ten women. In a 100-mile race there was minimal difference in the average time taken to finish or the speed of the males and females at the front of the race. Any difference had essentially shrunk to one to three per cent. This narrowing of the gap is where standout performances from top athletes such as Herron or Jasmin Paris can translate to a win on the day.

A win that comes from a lifetime of training and preparation. Of planning and working hard when things get tough. Paris is competitive by nature, but her ultra career has never been about competing with men. She had never thought that her abilities might differ from those of the male ultra runners she competes with, including her husband, Konrad Rawlik. After finishing the Barkley, she said: 'The fact that I was a woman wasn't in any way a barrier in my mind. But I'm incredibly happy to be able to inspire women and girls in sport. I also hope maybe it encourages people to have some hobbies of their own when kids, work and life get in the way. Because it has certainly been really good for my mental health.' A petition to add Paris' name to the shortlist for BBC Sports Personality of the Year gathered 15,000 signatures in a short space of time. It led to an invitation to start the women's race at the London Marathon. Many who would normally have no interest in endurance sport now know who she is and have indeed been inspired.

...

One common theme of the women in this book is curiosity. They wanted to see if they could. Often they wanted an adventure. Sometimes they needed something just for themselves. If they won outright, broke a record or became the first to do something, that was the icing on the cake. So many of them lift up and support other women along the way, whether as a role model, mentor, coach or through organisations such as SheRACES. They are not doing it for the limelight; for many that is an uncomfortable side effect. Nonetheless, it does give them a platform to talk about the things they care about, whether that's girls in sport, being active, sustainability, mental health, motherhood, menopause, or a plethora of other topics. They look to the future and when one challenge is done, they know there will be another around the corner.

In order for more women to reach their full potential we need to stop thinking of them as an afterthought. It hardly needs to be said, yet it does: female athletes should not be secondary to men. We need to build confidence that women belong on the start line. The media have a duty to ensure female visibility in the ultra-sport community and to celebrate achievements on an equal standing. But perhaps most importantly, we need to far better understand the role of female physiology in endurance. This will enable us to identify the advantages in muscle make-up, metabolism, and fatigue. It will enable the development of evidence-based training plans that suit women's needs rather than relying on trial and error. With greater knowledge, sports scientists can produce guidance that reflects a woman's life course through menstruation, pregnancy and menopause. Deeper insight into the science of endurance will actually help all athletes, male or female. Understanding how to best use sleep deprivation, pacing, and psychological strategies to their full advantage is something that benefits all endurance athletes. Listening to women who have learned what works for them is a good starting point. Having reviewed all the evidence and seen repeated patterns throughout history around the barriers to entry, limited expectations and lack of understanding of female endurance potential, we are ending our investigation by making a call to action. You can see our manifesto on the next page.

While it is a tempting proposition to ask whether women are faster in the long run, perhaps that is the wrong question. We are falling into the trap of judging women against the baseline of what men can achieve. Instead, let us celebrate female ultra achievement on its own terms. Let us see what women are capable of when we are fully supported to be the best version of ourselves. As a society, we need to tear down the dominant sexist narrative and enable women to go beyond expectations, set daunting challenges and take meaningful adventures. To help women become unstoppable.

OUR MANIFESTO FOR CHANGE

W e need to do more to ensure that women can fulfil their potential in endurance events. So we are ending our investigation by making a call to action. We want to see:

- **Female-specific sport endurance research.** Women have to be included in studies in far greater numbers and those studies must follow best practice on evaluating sex-based differences. The framework for inclusion of more women in well-executed sport and exercise research already exists. An international team of researchers led by Kirsty Elliott-Sale at Manchester Metropolitan University set out the standards of practice in 2021 (see Notes). Now researchers must use them. Moreover, universities, funding bodies, ethics committees and journals should require that researchers adhere to these standards when awarding grants and publishing studies.

- **Female-specific training guidelines**. Recommendations for training for ultra races are published by the events themselves, by coaches, and by specialist magazines, books and websites.

The vast majority of the time, they all expect men and women to follow the same plan. Women have repeatedly told us that this leads to overtraining and injury, among other problems. One review in 2023 found that, if they could be determined from the evidence, sex-specific guidelines could have a 'significant impact' on the performance and health of female ultra runners. In addition, training guidelines for women should be informed by better research on such issues as strength and conditioning, menstruation, nutrition and recovery.

- **Kit designed for women.** From trainers to sports bras, technical equipment to comfortable clothing, female athletes should be able to wear kit that supports their endeavours rather than having to make do. All sportswear brands selling to women should produce kit specifically designed by, with and for women. (Just marketing the same kit in pink does not count.)

- **Equal media coverage and commentary.** In the 21st Century, this should go without saying, but: visibility in sport remains a big problem. All media organisations and events should commit to parity of coverage between men and women and set out how they plan to achieve this within a stated timeframe. Media organisations should pay attention to the language they use in their coverage. When they are called out on their record, they should actively listen and provide a clear, non-defensive response.

- **Equal prize money and sponsorship.** This should be a commitment from all events as standard, not just those positioning themselves as a female-friendly race or company. Fair maternity policies should also be in place for sponsored or funded athletes. UK Sport has issued guidance on the duty of care owed to athletes during and after pregnancy, as have some others.

- **SheRACES inclusivity guidelines at all races.** There has been welcome progress on this front, but there is still so much more that can be done to get women on the starting line. Not just with a photo of a female athlete on an event website, but embracing the full recommendations set out by SheRACES.

NOTES

In writing this book we drew upon a vast array of resources including interviews, peer-reviewed journal articles, conference presentations, reports, books, podcasts, news stories and first-person blogs. We spoke to more than 70 experts and read hundreds of research papers.

Here is a selection of the key papers and references we used, so you can delve deeper into the subject.

Chapter 1

Paris, Jasmin, 2019 Spine Race Blog https://jasminfellrunner.blogspot.com/2020/01/spine-race.html

Chapter 2

Hadgraft, Rob, 2022, Pioneers in Bloomers: The True Story of the Pedestriennes - British Sport's First Female Celebrities

Playing Pasts: The Online Magazine for Sports and Leisure History https://www.playingpasts.co.uk/author/dmartin/

Run Young 50: Women's running history and the stories of older runners https://runyoung50.co.uk/

Mortimer, Gavin, 2008, The Great Swim: The Epic Struggle to be The First Woman to Conquer the Channel

Hewitt, Rachel, 2024, In Her Nature, How Women Break Boundaries in the Great Outdoors

Chapter 3

Olympic History: From Ancient Greek Olympics to Modern Olympic Games https://olympics.com/ioc/ancient-olympic-games/history

Switzer, Kathine, 2009, Marathon Woman: Running the Race to Revolutionize Women's Sports

Hargreaves, Jennifer, 1994, Sporting Females : Critical Issues in the History and Sociology of Women's Sport

Guiberteau, Oliver, 2023, Bobbi Gibb: The Boston Marathon pioneer who raced a lie https://www.bbc.co.uk/sport/athletics/66615089

Lovesey, Peter, 2021, The forgotten first lady: Rediscovering Violet Piercy, marathon pioneer https://www.playingpasts.co.uk/articles/gender-and-sport/the-forgotten-first-ladyrediscovering-violet-piercy-marathon-pioneerpart-3/

Carroll, John, 2019, A history of women's running https://www.runnersworld.com/uk/training/motivation/a26748147/a-history-of-womens-running/

Tarasouleas, Athanasios, 1997, Stamata Revithi, "Alias Melpomeni" https://library.olympics.com/Default/doc/SYRACUSE/353009/stamata-revithi-alias-melpomeni-by-athanasios-tarasouleas?_lg=en-GB

Sears, Edward S, 2015, Running Through the Ages, 2nd Ed

Holmes, Katie, Women's marathon history – the 1960s https://runyoung50.co.uk/womens-marathon-history-1960s/

History of the Olympic Games https://www.history.com/topics/sports/olympic-games

Chapter 4

Holmes, Katie, 2022, Eleanor Adams and the first Spartathlon https://runyoung50.co.uk/the-first-spartathlon/

Kostman, Chris, 1988, The Year Badwater Became a Race https://www.badwater.com/blog/1987-the-year-badwater-became-a-race/

Ohly, Shane, 1992, Twenty years later - An interview with Helene Whitaker and Martin Stone https://www.dragonsbackrace.com/news/2012/3/7/twenty-years-later-an-interview-with-helene-whitaker-and-martin-stone

Chlouber, Cole, Leadville Race Series History: The Unforgettable Story of the Tarahumara and Ann Trason https://www.leadvilleraceseries.com/5017-2/

McDougall, Christopher, 2010, Born to Run: The Hidden Tribe, the Ultra-runners, and the Greatest Race the World has Never Seen

Tough Girl Podcast, 2016, Interview with Ann Trason

Chapter 5

Anstiss, Sue, 2021, Game On: The Unstoppable Rise of Women's Sport

Women in Sport, Research and Insights reports https://womeninsport.org/explore-the-issues/our-research-and-insights/

Women's Trail Running Fund, Here For The Women's Race campaign https://www.hereforthewomensrace.com/

Chapter 6

Run Equal campaign https://runequal.org/

Women's Sports Foundation, Research reports https://www.womenssportsfoundation.org/what-we-do/wsf-research/

Valentin, Stephanie, et al. 2021, Enablers and barriers in ultra-running: a comparison of male and female ultra-runners. Sport in Society, 25 (11): 2193–2212. https://doi.org/10.1080/17430437.2021.1898590

DUV Ultra Marathon Statistics https://statistik.d-u-v.org/

Run Repeat, The State of Ultra Running 2020 https://runrepeat.com/uk/state-of-ultra-running#key-results

Motevalli Mohamad, et al. 2022, Sex Differences in Racing History of Recreational 10 km to Ultra Runners. International Journal of Environmental Research and Public Health, 19 (20): 13291. https://doi.org/10.3390/ijerph192013291

Hutchinson, Alex, 2018, Endure: Mind, Body and the Curiously Elastic Limits of Human Performance

Chapter 7

Cochrane, Andy, 2024, 'I'm motivated by the puzzle': how Courtney Dauwalter became ultrarunning's GOAT https://www.theguardian.com/sport/2024/sep/25/courtney-dauwalter-ultrarunner-greatest

Ryan, Patrick, 2023, Courtney Dauwalter secures historic treble with UTMB 2023 victory https://run247.com/running-news/trail/utmb-2023-results-women-courtney-dauwalter-triple-crown-treble-history

Guiberteau, Oliver, 2024, Courtney Dauwalter: Step inside the 'pain cave', where rules are remade https://www.bbc.co.uk/sport/athletics/67945344

Ronto, Paul and Nikolova, Vania, 2020, The State of Ultra Running 2020 https://runrepeat.com/uk/state-of-ultra-running

Whipp, Brian and Ward, Susana, 1992, Will women soon outrun men? Nature, 355: 25

O Deaner, Robert, et al, 2016, Men are More Likely than Women to Slow in the Marathon. Medicine & Science in Sports & Exercise, 47(3): 607–616

Hunter, Sandra K, et al, 2023, The Biological Basis of Sex Differences in Athletic Performance: Consensus Statement for the American College of Sports Medicine. Translational Journal of the ACSM, 8 (4): 1-33

Tiller, Nicholas B, et al, 2021, Do Sex Differences in Physiology Confer a Female Advantage in Ultra-Endurance Sport? Sports Medicine, 51 (5): 895-915

Tiller, Nicolas B, et al, 2022, Sex-Specific Physiological Responses to Ultramarathon. Medicine & Science in Sports & Exercise, 54(10): 1647-1656

Yu, Christine, 2023, Up to Speed: The Groundbreaking Science of Women Athletes

Chapter 8

Illidi, Camilla R and Jensen, Dennis, 2004, Effects of Sports Bras and Breast Volume on Pulmonary System and Respiratory Symptom Responses to Exercise in Healthy Females. Medicine & Science in Sports & Exercise, Published online Sep 16. doi: 10.1249/MSS.0000000000003561

Bastone, Kelly, 2017, A Brief History of the Sports Bra https://www.runnersworld.com/runners-stories/a20860634/a-brief-history-of-the-sports-bra/

Cowley, Emma S, et al, 2021, "Invisible Sportswomen": The Sex Data Gap in Sport and Exercise Science Research. Women in Sport and Physical Activity Journal, 29 (2): 1-6

Cowley, Emma S, et al, 2023, "Invisible Sportswomen 2.0"—Digging Deeper Into Gender Bias in Sport and Exercise Science Research: Author Gender, Editorial Board Gender, and Research Quality. Women in Sport and Physical Activity Journal, 32 (3): 1-8

Smith, Ella S and Burke, Louise M, 2024, Have We Considered Women in Current Sports Nutrition Guidelines? Nutrition Today 59 (4): 168-176

De Koning, Jos J and Foster Carl, 2024, Standing on the Shoulders of Giants: Essential Papers in Sports and Exercise Physiology. International Journal of Sports Physiology and Performance, 19 (8): 841–845

Elliott-Sale, Kirsty et al, 2021. Methodological Considerations for Studies in Sport and Exercise Science with Women as Participants: A Working Guide for Standards of Practice for Research on Women. Sports Medicine. 2021, 51(5): 843-861

Chapter 9

Lacy, Sarah and Ocobock, Cara, 2023, Woman the hunter: The archaeological evidence. American Anthropologist, 1-13

Ocobock, Cara and Lacy, Sarah, 2023, Woman the hunter: The physiological evidence. American Anthropologist, 1–12

Ocobock, Cara and Lacy, Sarah, 2023, The Theory That Men Evolved to Hunt and Women Evolved to Gather Is Wrong https://www.scientificamerican.com/article/the-theory-that-men-evolved-to-hunt-and-women-evolved-to-gather-is-wrong1/

Bohannon, Cat, 2023, Eve: How The Female Body Drove 200 Million Years of Human Evolution

Chapter 10

Hunter, Sandra K, 2016, The Relevance of Sex Differences in Performance Fatigability. Medicine & Science in Sports & Exercise, 48 (11): 2247-2256

Le Mat, Franck, et al, 2023, Running Endurance in Women Compared to Men: Retrospective Analysis of Matched Real-World Big Data. Sports Medicine, 53 (4):917-926

Besson, Thibault, et al, 2022, Sex Differences in Endurance Running. Sports Medicine, 52: 1235–1257

Chapter 11

Cox, Lynne, 2016, Swimming in the Sink: An Episode of the Heart

Eichenberger, Evelyn, Knechtle, Beat, et al. 2012. Best performances by men and women open-water swimmers during the 'English Channel Swim' from 1900 to 2010. Journal of Sports Sciences, 30 (12): 1295–1301. https://doi.org/10.1080/02640414.2012.709264

Knechtle, Beat, et al. 2015. Women cross the 'Catalina Channel' faster than men. SpringerPlus 4, 332. https://doi.org/10.1186/s40064-015-1086-4

Hamadeh, Mazen, et al. 2005. Estrogen Supplementation Reduces Whole Body Leucine and Carbohydrate Oxidation and Increases Lipid Oxidation in Men during Endurance Exercise, The Journal of Clinical Endocrinology & Metabolism, 90 (6): 3592–3599. https://doi.org/10.1210/jc.2004-1743

Chapter 12

Futterman, Matthew, 2023, Chelsea Sodaro Conquered Kona. Then the Real Struggles Returned https://www.nytimes.com/2023/03/30/sports/ironwoman-kona-chelsea-sodaro.html

Jackson, Mia, 2019, Athlete mothers pushing scientific, cultural change https://globalsportmatters.com/health/2019/12/02/athlete-mothers-pushing-scientific-cultural-change/

Carmichael, Ryanne, Considerations for the Pregnant Endurance Athlete. Strength and Conditioning Journal 43 (6): 35-4

Goom, Tom, Donnelly, Gráinne and Brockwell, Emma, 2019, Returning to running postnatal – guidelines for medical, health and fitness professionals managing this population https://absolute.physio/wp-content/uploads/2019/09/returning-to-running-postnatal-guidelines.pdf

Darroch, Francine E, et al, Running from responsibility: athletic governing bodies, corporate sponsors, and the failure to support pregnant and postpartum elite female distance runners. Sport in Society, 22(12): 2141–2160

Darroch, Francine E, et al, 2023, Effect of Pregnancy in 42 Elite to World-Class Runners on Training and Performance Outcomes. Medicine & Science in Sports & Exercise, 55 (1): 93-100

Meijen, Carla, 2023, Empowered Birth: Lessons from Sport Psychology for Your Maternity Journey

Thurber, Caitlin, et al, 2019, Extreme events reveal an alimentary limit on sustained maximal human energy expenditure. Science Advances, 5 (6): eaaw0341. doi: 10.1126/sciadv.aaw0341

American College of Obstetricians and Gynecologists, Guidance on Exercise in Pregnancy https://www.acog.org/womens-health/faqs/exercise-during-pregnancy

Claibourne, Alex, Jevtovic, Filip and May, Linda E, 2023, A narrative review of exercise dose during pregnancy. Birth Defects Research, 115 (17): 1581-1597

Chapter 13

The Sleep Foundation, Women and sleep. https://www.sleepfoundation.org/women-sleep

White, Caleb, 2023, Women More Resilient to Sleep Deprivation Than Men Due to Their Sex Hormones https://www.sciencetimes.com/articles/47061/20231113/women-more-resilient-sleep-deprivation-men-due-sex-hormones-study.htm

Mong, Jessica A and Cusmano, Danielle M, 2016, Sex differences in sleep: impact of biological sex and sex steroids. Philosophical Transactions of the Royal Society B: 371

Lok, Renske, Qian, Jingyi and Chellappa, Sarah L, 2024, Sex differences in sleep, circadian rhythms, and metabolism: Implications for precision medicine. Sleep Medicine Reviews, 75: 101926. doi: 10.1016/j.smrv.2024.101926

Diary of a CEO podcast with Stephen Bartlett. The Woman Who Helps Athletes Sleep. August 2024

Chapter 14

Verjee, Sabrina, 2022, Where There's a Hill: One woman, 214 Lake District fells, four attempts, one record-breaking Wainwrights run

RunRepeat, 2023, Women are Better Runners than Men https://runrepeat.com/uk/research-women-are-better-runners-than-men

Deaner, Robert, et al, 2015. Men are more likely than women to slow in the marathon. Medicine & Science in Sports & Exercise, 47 (3): 607-16.

Chapter 15

Srikanth, Ryal,i et al, 2024, Deep learning models reveal replicable, generalizable, and behaviorly relevant sex differences in human functional brain organization. Proceedings of the National Academy of Sciences, 121 (9) https://doi.org/10.1073/pnas.2310012121

Nicholls, Adam et al, 2007, Stressors, coping, and coping effectiveness: Gender, type of sport, and skill differences. Journal of Sports Sciences, 25 (13), 1521–1530. https://doi.org/10.1080/02640410701230479

Cycling Europe podcast, episode 30, Tandem WOW / Joff Summerfield

Chapter 16

Danielle Wilson, et al. 2019, "The zipper effect": Exploring the interrelationship of mental toughness and self-compassion among Canadian elite women athletes. Psychology of Sport and Exercise, 40: 61-70. https://doi.org/10.1016/j.psychsport.2018.09.006

Taylor, Shelley, et al. 2000, Biobehavioral responses to stress in females: tend-and-befriend, not fight-or-flight. Psychological Review, 107 (3): 411-29.

Chapter 17

Mimi Anderson and Lucy Waterlow, 2017, Beyond Impossible

Romer Tobias, et al, 2014, Age and ultra-marathon performance - 50 to 1,000 km distances from 1969 - 2012. Springerplus 25 (3):693.

Abou Shoak, et al, 2013, Participation and performance trends in ultracycling. Journal of Sports Medicine 4:41-51. https://doi.org/10.2147/OAJSM.S40142

Chapter 18

SheRACES https://www.sheraces.com/

Adidas Safety Survey, 2023, https://news.adidas.com/running/new-adidas-study-finds-92--of-women-are-concerned-for-their-safety-when-they-go-for-a-run/s/c318f69e-7575-4ced-bbf3-9db6d2ab1642

Teranishi Martinez C, et al, 2023, Sexual Harassment and Assault across Trail and Ultrarunning Communities: A Mixed-Method Study Exploring Gender Differences. Social Sciences 12 (6): 359. https://doi.org/10.3390/socsci12060359

Chapter 19

Stacy Sims with Selene Yeager, 2016, ROAR: Match your food and fitness to your unique female physiology for optimum performance, great health, and a strong body for life

Renee McGregor, 2022, More Fuel You: Understanding your body & how to fuel your adventures

Elliott-Sale, Kirsty and Pitchers, Guy. 2019. Considerations for coaches training female athletes. Professional Strength & Conditioning 55: 19-30.

Folscher, Lindy-Lee, et al. 2015, Ultra-Marathon Athletes at Risk for the Female Athlete Triad. Sports Medicine - Open 1, 29. https://doi.org/10.1186/s40798-015-0027-7

Chapter 20

Angie Brown, 2024, Jasmin Paris first woman to complete gruelling Barkley Marathons race https://www.bbc.co.uk/news/uk-scotland-edinburgh-east-fife-68643341

DUV Ultra Marathon Statistics https://statistik.d-u-v.org/

Mitchell, Melanie, 2024, Lululemon is Pushing the Boundaries for Female Athletes by Launching 'FURTHER' https://run.outsideonline.com/road/road-culture/lululemon-female-athletes-launches-further/

McCleery J, Diamond E, Kelly R, et al, 2024, Centering the female athlete voice in a sports science research agenda: a modified Delphi survey with Team USA athletes. British Journal of Sports Medicine, 58: 1107-1114

Tiller, Nicholas B and Illidi, Camilla R, 2024, Sex differences in ultramarathon performance in races with comparable numbers of males and females. Applied Physiology, Nutrition, and Metabolism, 49 (8): 1129-1136

Manifesto

Elliott-Sale, Kirsty et al, 2021. Methodological Considerations for Studies in Sport and Exercise Science with Women as Participants: A Working Guide for Standards of Practice for Research on Women. Sports Medicine. 2021, 51(5): 843-861

Kelly, Claudia, 2023, Is There Evidence for the Development of Sex-Specific Guidelines for Ultramarathon Coaches and Athletes? A Systematic Review. Sports Medicine Open, 9: 6

UK Sport, 2023, Pregnancy Guidelines. https://www.uksport.gov.uk/resources/pregnancy-guidance

SheRaces Race Guidelines https://www.sheraces.com/race-guidelines

ACKNOWLEDGEMENTS

Back in 2001, we were two naive postgraduate students meeting for the first time on a journalism masters at the University of Sheffield, in northern England. After a year we disappeared into industry and loosely kept in touch. Almost two decades later, we found our lives overlapping once more. By this point, we were both freelance journalists and mums to small children. Individually, we used running as a form of escapism to give us head space from the chaos of work and family life. By 2019, we were both beginning to explore the world of ultra running and despite living 100 miles apart we met up at races or set off on our own adventures. During these long runs, which could last for a whole weekend, we talked about our aspirations as runners, journalists and mothers. We chewed over potential book topics and machinated on our frustration at the male gaze in sport – and publishing.

There were many literal and metaphorical twists in the trail along the way, but our final destination was this book. It has morphed from an initial seed planted by an editor, Matt Lowing, who was the first to champion a female viewpoint. We will always be grateful to him for believing in this story, when others in the publishing world said it was not a marketable book because 'men wouldn't buy it.' Fortunately,

Martin Hickman at Canbury Press was not one of these naysayers. He understood that women had their own story to tell and it was time to shake up the status quo. His guidance and support have helped immeasurably in shaping this book into something we believe both women and men will enjoy. We acknowledge the irony that it took a man to say 'yes', when female marketers said 'no.'

For the past two years we have been consumed by the research and writing of this book. It was difficult to know where to start. We had a spreadsheet filled with hundreds of links to research papers and news articles, and our phones were filled with podcast downloads. It was all a little overwhelming. So we began by talking to women at the heart of this story. We reached out to athletes worldwide who were generous with their time and candid with their responses. Top of the list is Jasmin Paris, one of the first elite athletes we interviewed. She sits in great company alongside Lynne Cox, Helene Whitaker, Sabrina Verjee, Sophie Power, Corrine Malcolm, Mimi Anderson, Vriko Kwok, Eleanor Baverstock, Catherine Dixon, Rachael Marsden, Del Lloyd, Kim Beckinsale, Jamie Aarons, Hannah Walsh, Jackie Kabler, Lael Cox, Eleanor Robinson, Wendy Dodds, Chelsea Sodaro and Stephanie Howe – who all shared their remarkable stories with immense humility. Many of these interviews would not have been possible without introductions from Damian Hall, to whom we owe the biggest pot of tea. Unfortunately, some of the amazing women we chatted to did not make the final pages, but their contribution undoubtedly helped to shape the narrative. So thank you to Beth Pascall, Jasmijn Muller, Katie Wright, Nicky Spinks, Alicia Christofi-Walshe, Nikki Love and Allie Bailey. The list of outstanding female endurance athletes is a long one and we couldn't cover them all but we see you and celebrate your success. Whilst in the throes of research we became acutely aware of those who came before us and the indomitable work of Christine Yu, Sue Anstiss, Alex Hutchinson, Helen Gorman, Lucy Waterlow, Rachel Hewitt and Marie Sammons.

Thank you for shedding light on endurance, sport and the power of women.

...

Paramount to this book was telling the first-hand experience of women in ultra-endurance sport. But anecdotal evidence is not enough. We wanted to truly understand what the empirical data said, and where the gaps in research lay. Our goal was to create as complete a picture as possible of the multifaceted reasons why women excel at ultra sport and the barriers placed in their way. For this we turned to the research community. We are indebted to all the sports scientists, psychologists, dieticians, sociologists, anthropologists and historians who were able to translate complex ideas into layperson language for two wide-eyed health journalists. Stacy Sims, Renee McGregor, Chantelle Murnaghan, Nick Tiller, Bethan Taylor-Swaine, Fiona Beddoes, Hans Degens, Martin Turner, Josephine Perry, Andrew Lane, David Collins, Samuele Marcora, Michelle Jeitler, Puck Alkemade, Margie Davenport, Martin Dean, Katie Holmes, Derek Martin, Sandra Hunter, Guillame Millet, Beat Knechtle, Nicky Keay, Camilla Illidi, Emma Cowley, Lewis James, Carla Meijen, Stephen Gonzalez, Cara Ocobock, Cat Bohannon, Herman Pontzer, Linda May, Ryanne Carmichael, Jessica Mong, Carissa Gardiner, Cheri Mah, Jason Koop - you all informed us with your depth of research and sound wisdom.

...

As cliche as it sounds, finishing this book has felt like an endurance feat in itself. Thousands of WhatsApp messages, emails and Discord chats have been exchanged between us. At times we felt our heads would explode as they filled up with conflicting evidence and we continually met gaping chasms in the research. We were simultaneously working full time as freelance journalists, often with far too much on our plates.

Throughout this whole process our families have also endured. Our partners have been extremely accommodating, especially in the final weeks when we had to disappear to the countryside together to finish the final edits. Mark Hoyle and Mark Dayman are the patient men behind the strong women. And finally, we mustn't forget our children. They have understood when mummy needed to put a Do Not Disturb sign on the door or had to escape for a four-hour run. So thank you to Byron, Ivor, Lucy, Sam and Henry. We are delighted that you all know who Jasmin Paris is.

...

As we have written this book, we have been grateful to the supportive women around us who have been excited to hear about our project and have willed us on. Our friends who run, swim, cycle and hike and always say yes to a challenge. To the women at Great Bowden Runners who continue to impress us with their blossoming confidence as they venture into the unknown. And to you, the reader, whoever you are, we hope you are as inspired by the adventures and spirit of the women in this book as we have been.

Lily Canter and Emma Wilkinson

ABOUT THE AUTHORS

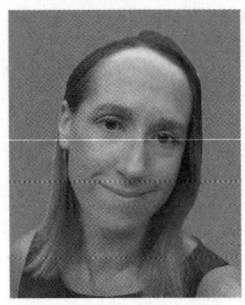 **Lily Canter** is a freelance running, fitness and adventure travel journalist writing for Runner's World, Live for the Outdoors, Women's Health, The Guardian and Metro. She is an England Athletics running coach and founder of women's only club Great Bowden Runners. She loves to spend her spare time competing in ultra marathons and canicrossing with her dog. Instagram: @lilycanter

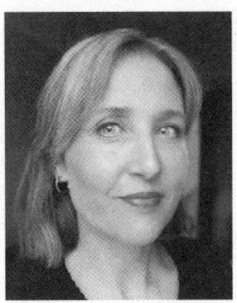 **Emma Wilkinson** is an award-winning freelance journalist specialising in medicine, science and health. She has written for the Sunday Times, BBC, Pulse, the BMJ and Lancet among others. Emma lives in Sheffield and runs up hills for fun. Instagram: @emmawjourno

More titles from Canbury Press

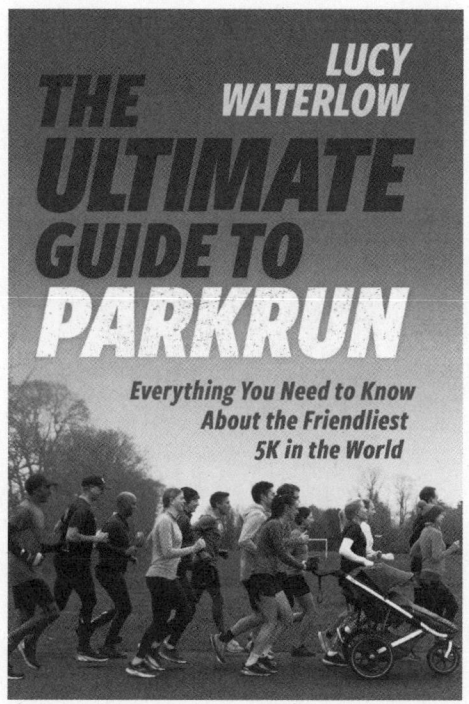

The Ultimate Guide to parkrun
Everything You Need to Know About the Friendliest 5K in
the World
Lucy Waterlow
ISBN: 9781914487361

'A brilliant emotive book which spreads the joy and love of
parkrun' — *Dame Kelly Holmes*

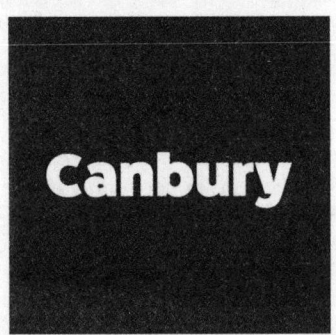

Are you an author?

Our aim is to depict the world as it really is, stripped of spin.

Modern non-fiction from London

www.canburypress.com

info@canburypress.com